Practice the HESI A2!

Health Information Systems
Practice Test Questions

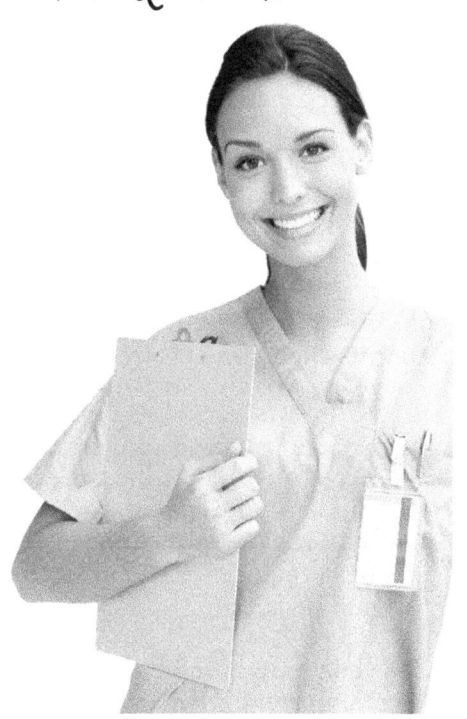

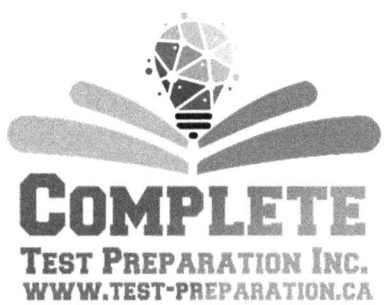

COMPLETE
TEST PREPARATION INC.
WWW.TEST-PREPARATION.CA

**We strongly recommend that students check with exam providers for up-to-date information regarding test content.**

ISBN-13: 978-1478311355
ISBN-10: 1478311355

Version 7.6 April 2019

Published by
Complete Test Preparation Inc.
Victoria BC Canada

Visit us on the web at https://www.test-preparation.ca
Printed in the USA

# About Complete Test Preparation Inc.

The Complete Test Preparation Team has been publishing high quality study materials since 2005. Over one million students visit our websites every year, and thousands of students, teachers and parents all over the world (over 100 countries) have purchased our teaching materials, curriculum, study guides and practice tests.

Complete Test Preparation is committed to providing students with the best study materials and practice tests available on the market. Members of our team combine years of teaching experience, with experienced writers and editors, all with advanced degrees.

## Feedback

We welcome your feedback.  Email us at feedback@test-preparation.ca with your comments and suggestions.   We carefully review all suggestions and often incorporate reader suggestions into upcoming versions. As a Print on Demand Publisher, we update our products frequently.

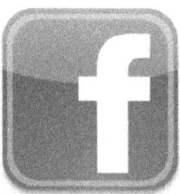

## Find us on Facebook

**www.facebook.com/CompleteTestPreparation**

# Contents

# Getting Started

CONGRATULATIONS! By deciding to take the Health Education Systems (HESI® A2) Exam, you have taken the first step toward a great future! Of course, there is no point in taking this important examination unless you intend to do your best to earn the highest grade you possibly can. That means getting yourself organized and discovering the best approaches, methods and strategies to master the material. Yes, that will require real effort and dedication but if you are willing to focus your energy and devote the study time necessary, before you know it you will be opening that letter of acceptance to the school of your dreams.

We know that taking on a new endeavour can be a little scary, and it is easy to feel unsure of where to begin. That's where we come in. This study guide is designed to help you improve your test-taking skills, show you a few tricks of the trade and increase both your competency and confidence.

## The Health Education Systems A2® Exam

The HESI® A2 exam is composed of modules and not all schools use all the modules. It is therefore very important that you find out what modules your school will use! That way you won't waste valuable study time learning something that isn't on your exam!

The HESI® A2 Modules are: Mathematics, Vocabulary, Reading Comprehension, English grammar, and a Science module which includes, Biology, Chemistry, Physics, Basic Scientific principles and Anatomy and Physiology.

You don`t have to worry because these sections are included in this study guide. However, to maximize your study time, it is very important to check which modules your university offers before studying everything under the sun!

While we seek to make our guide as comprehensive as possible, note that like all entrance exams, the HESI® A2 Exam might be adjusted at some future point. New material might be added, or content that is no longer relevant or applicable might be removed. It is always a good idea to give the materials you receive when you register to take the HESI® a careful review.

# The HESI® Study Plan

Now that you have made the decision to take the HESI, it's time to get started. Before you do another thing, you will need to figure out a plan of attack. The best study tip is to start early! The longer the time period you devote to regular study practice, the more likely you will retain the material and be able to reach it quickly. If you thought that 1x20 is the same as 2x10, guess what? It really is not, when it comes to study time. Reviewing material for just an hour per day over the course of 20 days is far better than studying for two hours a day for only 10 days. The more often you revisit a particular piece of information, the better you will know it. Not only will your grasp and understanding be better, but your ability to reach into your brain and quickly and efficiently pull out the tidbit you need, will be greatly enhanced as well.

The great Chinese scholar and philosopher Confucius believed that true knowledge could be defined as knowing what you know and what you do not know. The first step in preparing for the HESI® Exam is to assess your strengths and weaknesses. You may already have an idea of what you know and what you do not know, but evaluating yourself using our Self-Assessment modules for each of the three areas, math, english science and reading, will clarify the details.

### Making a Study Schedule

To make your study time the most productive, you will need to develop a study plan. The purpose of the plan is to organize all the bits of pieces of information in such a way that you will not feel overwhelmed. Rome was not built in a day, and learning everything you will need to know to pass the HESI® Exam is going to take time, too. Arranging the material you need to learn into manageable chunks is the best way to go. Each study session should make you feel as though you have accomplished your goal, and your goal is simply to learn what you planned to learn during that particular session. Try to organize the content in such a way that each study session builds on previous ones. That way, you will retain the information, be better able to reach it, and review the previous bits and pieces at the same time.

## Self-assessment

**The Best Study Tip!** The best study tip is to start early! The longer you study regularly, the more you will retain and 'learn' the material. Studying for 1 hour per day for 20 days is far better than studying for 2 hours for 10 days.

### What don't you know?

The first step is to assess your strengths and weaknesses. You may already have an idea of where your weaknesses are, or you can take our Self-assessment modules for each of the areas, math, English, science and reading.

Below is a table to assess your exam readiness in each content area. You can fill this in now, and correct if necessary after completing the self-assessments, or fill it in after you have taken the self-assessments.

## Self-assessment

**The Best Study Tip!** The best study tip is to start early! The longer you study regularly, the more you will retain and 'learn' the material. Studying for 1 hour per day for 20 days is far better than studying for 2 hours for 10 days.

**What don't you know?**

The first step is to assess your strengths and weaknesses. You may already have an idea of where your weaknesses are, or you can take our Self-assessment modules for each of the areas, Math, English, Science and Reading Comprehension.

| Exam Component | Rate 1 to 5 |
|---|---|
| **Reading Comprehension** | |
| | |
| Paragraph & Passage Comprehension | |
| Drawing inferences & conclusions | |
| **English Grammar** | |
| **Vocabulary** | |
| | |
| **Math** | |
| Fractions | |
| Decimals | |
| Percent | |
| Word Problems | |
| Basic Algebra | |
| **Science** | |
| Anatomy and Physiology | |
| Biology | |
| Chemistry | |

# Making a Study Schedule

The key to making a study plan is to divide the material you need to learn into manageable size and learn it, while at the same time reviewing the material that you already know.

Using the table above, any scores of 3 or below, you need to spend time learning, reviewing and practicing this subject area. A score of 4 means you need to review the material, but you don't have to spend time re-learning. A score of 5 and you are OK with just an occasional review before the exam.

A score of 0 or 1 means you really need to work on this area and should allocate the most time and the highest priority. Some students prefer a 5-day plan and others a 10-day plan. It also depends on how much time until the exam.

Here is an example of a 5-day plan based on an example from the table above:

**Fractions:** 1  Study 1 hour everyday – review on last day
**Biology:** 3  Study 1 hour for 2 days then ½ hour a day, then review
**Vocabulary:** 4  Review every second day
**Word Problems:** 2 Study 1 hour on the first day – then ½ hour everyday
**Reading Comprehension:** 5  Review for ½ hour every other day
**Algebra:** 5  Review for ½ hour every other day
**Chemistry:** 5 very confident – review a few times.

Using this example, Chemistry and Grammar are good and only need occasional review. Biology is also good and needs 'some' review. Decimals need a bit of work, Word Problems need a lot of work and Fractions are very weak and need the majority of time. Based on this, here is a sample study plan:

| Day | Subject | Time |
|---|---|---|
| | | |
| **Monday** | | |
| Study | Fractions | 1 hour |
| Study | Word Problems | 1 hour |
| | **½ hour break** | |
| Study | Biology | 1 hour |
| Review | Chemistry | ½ hour |
| | | |
| **Tuesday** | | |
| Study | Fractions | 1 hour |
| Study | Word Problems | ½ hour |
| | **½ hour break** | |
| Study | Decimals | ½ hour |
| Review | Vocabulary | ½ hour |
| Review | Grammar | ½ hour |
| | | |
| **Wednesday** | | |
| Study | Fractions | 1 hour |
| Study | Word Problems | ½ hour |
| | **½ hour break** | |
| Study | Biology | ½ hour |
| Review | Chemistry | ½ hour |
| | | |
| **Thursday** | | |
| Study | Fractions | ½ hour |
| Study | Word Problems | ½ hour |
| Review | Biology | ½ hour |
| | **½ hour break** | |
| Review | Grammar | ½ hour |
| Review | Vocabulary | ½ hour |

| | | |
|---|---|---|
| **Friday** | | |
| Review | Fractions | ½ hour |
| Review | Word Problems | ½ hour |
| Review | Biology | ½ hour |
| | **½ hour break** | |
| Review | Vocabulary | ½ hour |
| Review | Grammar | ½ hour |

# Practice Test Questions Set 1

## Section I – Reading Comprehension

**Questions:** 35
**Time:** 60 Minutes

## Section II – Mathematics

**Questions:** 50
**Time:** 60 Minutes

## Section III English Grammar

**Questions:** 50
**Time:** 50 Minutes

## Section IV - Vocabulary

**Questions:** 50
**Time:** 50 Minutes

## Section V – Part I – Science

**Questions:** 75
**Time:** 125 minutes

## Section VI Anatomy & Physiology

**Questions:** 25
**Time:** 25 minutes

The questions below are not the same as you will find on the HESI® - that would be too easy! And nobody knows what the questions will be and they change all the time. Below are general questions that cover the same subject areas as the HESI.  While the format and exact wording of the questions may differ slightly, and change from year to year, if you can answer the questions below, you will have no problem with the HESI.

For the best results, take this Practice Test as if it were the real exam. Set aside time when you will not be disturbed, and a location that is quiet and free of distractions. Read the instructions carefully, read each question carefully, and answer to the best of your ability.

Use the bubble answer sheets provided. When you have completed the Practice Test, check your answer against the Answer Key and read the explanation provided.

Do not attempt more than one set of practice test questions in one day.  After completing the first practice test, wait two or three days before attempting the second set of questions.

**This set of practice test questions contains all the HESI® modules.  Different schools use different modules so be sure to check with your school for the modules being used.**

# Reading Comprehension

|      | A | B | C | D | E |      | A | B | C | D | E |
|------|---|---|---|---|---|------|---|---|---|---|---|
| 1    | ○ | ○ | ○ | ○ | ○ | 21   | ○ | ○ | ○ | ○ | ○ |
| 2    | ○ | ○ | ○ | ○ | ○ | 22   | ○ | ○ | ○ | ○ | ○ |
| 3    | ○ | ○ | ○ | ○ | ○ | 23   | ○ | ○ | ○ | ○ | ○ |
| 4    | ○ | ○ | ○ | ○ | ○ | 24   | ○ | ○ | ○ | ○ | ○ |
| 5    | ○ | ○ | ○ | ○ | ○ | 25   | ○ | ○ | ○ | ○ | ○ |
| 6    | ○ | ○ | ○ | ○ | ○ | 26   | ○ | ○ | ○ | ○ | ○ |
| 7    | ○ | ○ | ○ | ○ | ○ | 27   | ○ | ○ | ○ | ○ | ○ |
| 8    | ○ | ○ | ○ | ○ | ○ | 28   | ○ | ○ | ○ | ○ | ○ |
| 9    | ○ | ○ | ○ | ○ | ○ | 29   | ○ | ○ | ○ | ○ | ○ |
| 10   | ○ | ○ | ○ | ○ | ○ | 30   | ○ | ○ | ○ | ○ | ○ |
| 11   | ○ | ○ | ○ | ○ | ○ | 31   | ○ | ○ | ○ | ○ | ○ |
| 12   | ○ | ○ | ○ | ○ | ○ | 32   | ○ | ○ | ○ | ○ | ○ |
| 13   | ○ | ○ | ○ | ○ | ○ | 33   | ○ | ○ | ○ | ○ | ○ |
| 14   | ○ | ○ | ○ | ○ | ○ | 34   | ○ | ○ | ○ | ○ | ○ |
| 15   | ○ | ○ | ○ | ○ | ○ | 35   | ○ | ○ | ○ | ○ | ○ |
| 16   | ○ | ○ | ○ | ○ | ○ |      |   |   |   |   |   |
| 17   | ○ | ○ | ○ | ○ | ○ |      |   |   |   |   |   |
| 18   | ○ | ○ | ○ | ○ | ○ |      |   |   |   |   |   |
| 19   | ○ | ○ | ○ | ○ | ○ |      |   |   |   |   |   |
| 20   | ○ | ○ | ○ | ○ | ○ |      |   |   |   |   |   |

# Mathematics

|     | A | B | C | D | E |     | A | B | C | D | E |
| --- | - | - | - | - | - | --- | - | - | - | - | - |
| 1 | ○ | ○ | ○ | ○ | ○ | 26 | ○ | ○ | ○ | ○ | ○ |
| 2 | ○ | ○ | ○ | ○ | ○ | 27 | ○ | ○ | ○ | ○ | ○ |
| 3 | ○ | ○ | ○ | ○ | ○ | 28 | ○ | ○ | ○ | ○ | ○ |
| 4 | ○ | ○ | ○ | ○ | ○ | 29 | ○ | ○ | ○ | ○ | ○ |
| 5 | ○ | ○ | ○ | ○ | ○ | 30 | ○ | ○ | ○ | ○ | ○ |
| 6 | ○ | ○ | ○ | ○ | ○ | 31 | ○ | ○ | ○ | ○ | ○ |
| 7 | ○ | ○ | ○ | ○ | ○ | 32 | ○ | ○ | ○ | ○ | ○ |
| 8 | ○ | ○ | ○ | ○ | ○ | 33 | ○ | ○ | ○ | ○ | ○ |
| 9 | ○ | ○ | ○ | ○ | ○ | 34 | ○ | ○ | ○ | ○ | ○ |
| 10 | ○ | ○ | ○ | ○ | ○ | 35 | ○ | ○ | ○ | ○ | ○ |
| 11 | ○ | ○ | ○ | ○ | ○ | 36 | ○ | ○ | ○ | ○ | ○ |
| 12 | ○ | ○ | ○ | ○ | ○ | 37 | ○ | ○ | ○ | ○ | ○ |
| 13 | ○ | ○ | ○ | ○ | ○ | 38 | ○ | ○ | ○ | ○ | ○ |
| 14 | ○ | ○ | ○ | ○ | ○ | 39 | ○ | ○ | ○ | ○ | ○ |
| 15 | ○ | ○ | ○ | ○ | ○ | 40 | ○ | ○ | ○ | ○ | ○ |
| 16 | ○ | ○ | ○ | ○ | ○ | 41 | ○ | ○ | ○ | ○ | ○ |
| 17 | ○ | ○ | ○ | ○ | ○ | 42 | ○ | ○ | ○ | ○ | ○ |
| 18 | ○ | ○ | ○ | ○ | ○ | 43 | ○ | ○ | ○ | ○ | ○ |
| 19 | ○ | ○ | ○ | ○ | ○ | 44 | ○ | ○ | ○ | ○ | ○ |
| 20 | ○ | ○ | ○ | ○ | ○ | 45 | ○ | ○ | ○ | ○ | ○ |
| 21 | ○ | ○ | ○ | ○ | ○ | 46 | ○ | ○ | ○ | ○ | ○ |
| 22 | ○ | ○ | ○ | ○ | ○ | 47 | ○ | ○ | ○ | ○ | ○ |
| 23 | ○ | ○ | ○ | ○ | ○ | 48 | ○ | ○ | ○ | ○ | ○ |
| 24 | ○ | ○ | ○ | ○ | ○ | 49 | ○ | ○ | ○ | ○ | ○ |
| 25 | ○ | ○ | ○ | ○ | ○ | 50 | ○ | ○ | ○ | ○ | ○ |

# English Grammar

| | A | B | C | D | E | | | A | B | C | D | E |
|---|---|---|---|---|---|---|---|---|---|---|---|---|
| 1 | ○ | ○ | ○ | ○ | ○ | | 26 | ○ | ○ | ○ | ○ | ○ |
| 2 | ○ | ○ | ○ | ○ | ○ | | 27 | ○ | ○ | ○ | ○ | ○ |
| 3 | ○ | ○ | ○ | ○ | ○ | | 28 | ○ | ○ | ○ | ○ | ○ |
| 4 | ○ | ○ | ○ | ○ | ○ | | 29 | ○ | ○ | ○ | ○ | ○ |
| 5 | ○ | ○ | ○ | ○ | ○ | | 30 | ○ | ○ | ○ | ○ | ○ |
| 6 | ○ | ○ | ○ | ○ | ○ | | 31 | ○ | ○ | ○ | ○ | ○ |
| 7 | ○ | ○ | ○ | ○ | ○ | | 32 | ○ | ○ | ○ | ○ | ○ |
| 8 | ○ | ○ | ○ | ○ | ○ | | 33 | ○ | ○ | ○ | ○ | ○ |
| 9 | ○ | ○ | ○ | ○ | ○ | | 34 | ○ | ○ | ○ | ○ | ○ |
| 10 | ○ | ○ | ○ | ○ | ○ | | 35 | ○ | ○ | ○ | ○ | ○ |
| 11 | ○ | ○ | ○ | ○ | ○ | | 36 | ○ | ○ | ○ | ○ | ○ |
| 12 | ○ | ○ | ○ | ○ | ○ | | 37 | ○ | ○ | ○ | ○ | ○ |
| 13 | ○ | ○ | ○ | ○ | ○ | | 38 | ○ | ○ | ○ | ○ | ○ |
| 14 | ○ | ○ | ○ | ○ | ○ | | 39 | ○ | ○ | ○ | ○ | ○ |
| 15 | ○ | ○ | ○ | ○ | ○ | | 40 | ○ | ○ | ○ | ○ | ○ |
| 16 | ○ | ○ | ○ | ○ | ○ | | 41 | ○ | ○ | ○ | ○ | ○ |
| 17 | ○ | ○ | ○ | ○ | ○ | | 42 | ○ | ○ | ○ | ○ | ○ |
| 18 | ○ | ○ | ○ | ○ | ○ | | 43 | ○ | ○ | ○ | ○ | ○ |
| 19 | ○ | ○ | ○ | ○ | ○ | | 44 | ○ | ○ | ○ | ○ | ○ |
| 20 | ○ | ○ | ○ | ○ | ○ | | 45 | ○ | ○ | ○ | ○ | ○ |
| 21 | ○ | ○ | ○ | ○ | ○ | | 46 | ○ | ○ | ○ | ○ | ○ |
| 22 | ○ | ○ | ○ | ○ | ○ | | 47 | ○ | ○ | ○ | ○ | ○ |
| 23 | ○ | ○ | ○ | ○ | ○ | | 48 | ○ | ○ | ○ | ○ | ○ |
| 24 | ○ | ○ | ○ | ○ | ○ | | 49 | ○ | ○ | ○ | ○ | ○ |
| 25 | ○ | ○ | ○ | ○ | ○ | | 50 | ○ | ○ | ○ | ○ | ○ |

# Vocabulary

|    | A | B | C | D | E |    |    | A | B | C | D | E |
|----|---|---|---|---|---|----|----|---|---|---|---|---|
| 1  | ○ | ○ | ○ | ○ | ○ |    | 26 | ○ | ○ | ○ | ○ | ○ |
| 2  | ○ | ○ | ○ | ○ | ○ |    | 27 | ○ | ○ | ○ | ○ | ○ |
| 3  | ○ | ○ | ○ | ○ | ○ |    | 28 | ○ | ○ | ○ | ○ | ○ |
| 4  | ○ | ○ | ○ | ○ | ○ |    | 29 | ○ | ○ | ○ | ○ | ○ |
| 5  | ○ | ○ | ○ | ○ | ○ |    | 30 | ○ | ○ | ○ | ○ | ○ |
| 6  | ○ | ○ | ○ | ○ | ○ |    | 31 | ○ | ○ | ○ | ○ | ○ |
| 7  | ○ | ○ | ○ | ○ | ○ |    | 32 | ○ | ○ | ○ | ○ | ○ |
| 8  | ○ | ○ | ○ | ○ | ○ |    | 33 | ○ | ○ | ○ | ○ | ○ |
| 9  | ○ | ○ | ○ | ○ | ○ |    | 34 | ○ | ○ | ○ | ○ | ○ |
| 10 | ○ | ○ | ○ | ○ | ○ |    | 35 | ○ | ○ | ○ | ○ | ○ |
| 11 | ○ | ○ | ○ | ○ | ○ |    | 36 | ○ | ○ | ○ | ○ | ○ |
| 12 | ○ | ○ | ○ | ○ | ○ |    | 37 | ○ | ○ | ○ | ○ | ○ |
| 13 | ○ | ○ | ○ | ○ | ○ |    | 38 | ○ | ○ | ○ | ○ | ○ |
| 14 | ○ | ○ | ○ | ○ | ○ |    | 39 | ○ | ○ | ○ | ○ | ○ |
| 15 | ○ | ○ | ○ | ○ | ○ |    | 40 | ○ | ○ | ○ | ○ | ○ |
| 16 | ○ | ○ | ○ | ○ | ○ |    | 41 | ○ | ○ | ○ | ○ | ○ |
| 17 | ○ | ○ | ○ | ○ | ○ |    | 42 | ○ | ○ | ○ | ○ | ○ |
| 18 | ○ | ○ | ○ | ○ | ○ |    | 43 | ○ | ○ | ○ | ○ | ○ |
| 19 | ○ | ○ | ○ | ○ | ○ |    | 44 | ○ | ○ | ○ | ○ | ○ |
| 20 | ○ | ○ | ○ | ○ | ○ |    | 45 | ○ | ○ | ○ | ○ | ○ |
| 21 | ○ | ○ | ○ | ○ | ○ |    | 46 | ○ | ○ | ○ | ○ | ○ |
| 22 | ○ | ○ | ○ | ○ | ○ |    | 47 | ○ | ○ | ○ | ○ | ○ |
| 23 | ○ | ○ | ○ | ○ | ○ |    | 48 | ○ | ○ | ○ | ○ | ○ |
| 24 | ○ | ○ | ○ | ○ | ○ |    | 49 | ○ | ○ | ○ | ○ | ○ |
| 25 | ○ | ○ | ○ | ○ | ○ |    | 50 | ○ | ○ | ○ | ○ | ○ |

# Science

| 1. Ⓐ Ⓑ Ⓒ Ⓓ | 21. Ⓐ Ⓑ Ⓒ Ⓓ | 41. Ⓐ Ⓑ Ⓒ Ⓓ | 61. Ⓐ Ⓑ Ⓒ Ⓓ |
|---|---|---|---|
| 2. Ⓐ Ⓑ Ⓒ Ⓓ | 22. Ⓐ Ⓑ Ⓒ Ⓓ | 42. Ⓐ Ⓑ Ⓒ Ⓓ | 62. Ⓐ Ⓑ Ⓒ Ⓓ |
| 3. Ⓐ Ⓑ Ⓒ Ⓓ | 23. Ⓐ Ⓑ Ⓒ Ⓓ | 43. Ⓐ Ⓑ Ⓒ Ⓓ | 63. Ⓐ Ⓑ Ⓒ Ⓓ |
| 4. Ⓐ Ⓑ Ⓒ Ⓓ | 24. Ⓐ Ⓑ Ⓒ Ⓓ | 44. Ⓐ Ⓑ Ⓒ Ⓓ | 64. Ⓐ Ⓑ Ⓒ Ⓓ |
| 5. Ⓐ Ⓑ Ⓒ Ⓓ | 25. Ⓐ Ⓑ Ⓒ Ⓓ | 45. Ⓐ Ⓑ Ⓒ Ⓓ | 65. Ⓐ Ⓑ Ⓒ Ⓓ |
| 6. Ⓐ Ⓑ Ⓒ Ⓓ | 26. Ⓐ Ⓑ Ⓒ Ⓓ | 46. Ⓐ Ⓑ Ⓒ Ⓓ | 66. Ⓐ Ⓑ Ⓒ Ⓓ |
| 7. Ⓐ Ⓑ Ⓒ Ⓓ | 27. Ⓐ Ⓑ Ⓒ Ⓓ | 47. Ⓐ Ⓑ Ⓒ Ⓓ | 67. Ⓐ Ⓑ Ⓒ Ⓓ |
| 8. Ⓐ Ⓑ Ⓒ Ⓓ | 28. Ⓐ Ⓑ Ⓒ Ⓓ | 48. Ⓐ Ⓑ Ⓒ Ⓓ | 68. Ⓐ Ⓑ Ⓒ Ⓓ |
| 9. Ⓐ Ⓑ Ⓒ Ⓓ | 29. Ⓐ Ⓑ Ⓒ Ⓓ | 49. Ⓐ Ⓑ Ⓒ Ⓓ | 69. Ⓐ Ⓑ Ⓒ Ⓓ |
| 10. Ⓐ Ⓑ Ⓒ Ⓓ | 30. Ⓐ Ⓑ Ⓒ Ⓓ | 50. Ⓐ Ⓑ Ⓒ Ⓓ | 70. Ⓐ Ⓑ Ⓒ Ⓓ |
| 11. Ⓐ Ⓑ Ⓒ Ⓓ | 31. Ⓐ Ⓑ Ⓒ Ⓓ | 51. Ⓐ Ⓑ Ⓒ Ⓓ | 71. Ⓐ Ⓑ Ⓒ Ⓓ |
| 12. Ⓐ Ⓑ Ⓒ Ⓓ | 32. Ⓐ Ⓑ Ⓒ Ⓓ | 52. Ⓐ Ⓑ Ⓒ Ⓓ | 72. Ⓐ Ⓑ Ⓒ Ⓓ |
| 13. Ⓐ Ⓑ Ⓒ Ⓓ | 33. Ⓐ Ⓑ Ⓒ Ⓓ | 53. Ⓐ Ⓑ Ⓒ Ⓓ | 73. Ⓐ Ⓑ Ⓒ Ⓓ |
| 14. Ⓐ Ⓑ Ⓒ Ⓓ | 34. Ⓐ Ⓑ Ⓒ Ⓓ | 54. Ⓐ Ⓑ Ⓒ Ⓓ | 74. Ⓐ Ⓑ Ⓒ Ⓓ |
| 15. Ⓐ Ⓑ Ⓒ Ⓓ | 35. Ⓐ Ⓑ Ⓒ Ⓓ | 55. Ⓐ Ⓑ Ⓒ Ⓓ | 75. Ⓐ Ⓑ Ⓒ Ⓓ |
| 16. Ⓐ Ⓑ Ⓒ Ⓓ | 36. Ⓐ Ⓑ Ⓒ Ⓓ | 56. Ⓐ Ⓑ Ⓒ Ⓓ | |
| 17. Ⓐ Ⓑ Ⓒ Ⓓ | 37. Ⓐ Ⓑ Ⓒ Ⓓ | 57. Ⓐ Ⓑ Ⓒ Ⓓ | |
| 18. Ⓐ Ⓑ Ⓒ Ⓓ | 38. Ⓐ Ⓑ Ⓒ Ⓓ | 58. Ⓐ Ⓑ Ⓒ Ⓓ | |
| 19. Ⓐ Ⓑ Ⓒ Ⓓ | 39. Ⓐ Ⓑ Ⓒ Ⓓ | 59. Ⓐ Ⓑ Ⓒ Ⓓ | |
| 20. Ⓐ Ⓑ Ⓒ Ⓓ | 40. Ⓐ Ⓑ Ⓒ Ⓓ | 60. Ⓐ Ⓑ Ⓒ Ⓓ | |

## Anatomy and Physiology

|    | A | B | C | D | E |    | A | B | C | D | E |
|----|---|---|---|---|---|----|---|---|---|---|---|
| 1  | ○ | ○ | ○ | ○ | ○ | 21 | ○ | ○ | ○ | ○ | ○ |
| 2  | ○ | ○ | ○ | ○ | ○ | 22 | ○ | ○ | ○ | ○ | ○ |
| 3  | ○ | ○ | ○ | ○ | ○ | 23 | ○ | ○ | ○ | ○ | ○ |
| 4  | ○ | ○ | ○ | ○ | ○ | 24 | ○ | ○ | ○ | ○ | ○ |
| 5  | ○ | ○ | ○ | ○ | ○ | 25 | ○ | ○ | ○ | ○ | ○ |
| 6  | ○ | ○ | ○ | ○ | ○ |    |   |   |   |   |   |
| 7  | ○ | ○ | ○ | ○ | ○ |    |   |   |   |   |   |
| 8  | ○ | ○ | ○ | ○ | ○ |    |   |   |   |   |   |
| 9  | ○ | ○ | ○ | ○ | ○ |    |   |   |   |   |   |
| 10 | ○ | ○ | ○ | ○ | ○ |    |   |   |   |   |   |
| 11 | ○ | ○ | ○ | ○ | ○ |    |   |   |   |   |   |
| 12 | ○ | ○ | ○ | ○ | ○ |    |   |   |   |   |   |
| 13 | ○ | ○ | ○ | ○ | ○ |    |   |   |   |   |   |
| 14 | ○ | ○ | ○ | ○ | ○ |    |   |   |   |   |   |
| 15 | ○ | ○ | ○ | ○ | ○ |    |   |   |   |   |   |
| 16 | ○ | ○ | ○ | ○ | ○ |    |   |   |   |   |   |
| 17 | ○ | ○ | ○ | ○ | ○ |    |   |   |   |   |   |
| 18 | ○ | ○ | ○ | ○ | ○ |    |   |   |   |   |   |
| 19 | ○ | ○ | ○ | ○ | ○ |    |   |   |   |   |   |
| 20 | ○ | ○ | ○ | ○ | ○ |    |   |   |   |   |   |

# Section I - Reading Comprehension

**Directions:** The following questions are based on several reading passages. Each passage is followed by a series of questions. Read each passage carefully, and then answer the questions based on it. You may reread the passage as often as you wish. When you have finished answering the questions based on one passage, go right onto the next passage. Choose the best answer based on the information given and implied.

**Questions 1 – 4 refer to the following passage.**

**Passage 1 - The Life of Helen Keller**

Many people have heard of Helen Keller. She is famous because she was unable to see or hear, but learned to speak and read and went onto attend college and earn a degree. Her life is a very interesting story, one that she developed into an autobiography, which was then adapted into both a stage play and a movie. How did Helen Keller overcome her disabilities to become a famous woman? Read onto find out.
Helen Keller was not born blind and deaf. When she was a small baby, she had a very high fever for several days. As a result of her sudden illness, baby Helen lost her eyesight and her hearing. Because she was so young when she went deaf and blind, Helen Keller never had any recollection of being able to see or hear. Since she could not hear, she could not learn to talk. Since she could not see, it was difficult for her to move around. For the first six years of her life, her world was very still and dark.

Imagine what Helen's childhood must have been like. She could not hear her mother's voice. She could not see the beauty of her parent's farm. She could not recognize who was giving her a hug, or a bath or even where her bedroom was each night. More sad, she could not communicate with her parents in any way. She could not express her feelings or tell them the things she wanted. It must have been a very sad childhood.

When Helen was six years old, her parents hired her a teacher named Anne Sullivan. Anne was a young woman who was almost blind. However, she could hear and she could read Braille, so she was a perfect teacher for young Helen. At first, Anne had a very hard time teaching Helen anything. She described her first impression of Helen as a "wild thing, not a child." Helen did not like Anne at first either. She bit and hit Anne when Anne tried to teach her. However, the two of them eventually came to have a great deal of love and respect.

Anne taught Helen to hear by putting her hands on people's throats. She could feel the sounds that people made. In time, Helen learned to feel what people said. Next, Anne taught Helen to read Braille, which is a way that books are written for the blind. Finally, Anne taught Helen to talk. Although Helen did learn to talk, it was hard for anyone but Anne to understand her.

As Helen grew older, more and more people were amazed by her story. She went to college and wrote books about her life. She gave talks to the public, with Anne at her side, translating her words. Today, both Anne Sullivan and Helen Keller are famous women who are respected for their lives' work.

**1. Helen Keller could not see and hear and so, what was her biggest problem in childhood?**

    a. Inability to communicate

    b. Inability to walk

    c. Inability to play

    d. Inability to eat

**2. Helen learned to hear by feeling the vibrations people made when they spoke. What were these vibrations were felt through?**

    a. Mouth

    b. Throat

    c. Ears

    d. Lips

## 3. From the passage, we can infer that Anne Sullivan was a patient teacher. We can infer this because

a. Helen hit and bit her and Anne still remained her teacher.

b. Anne taught Helen to read only.

c. Anne was hard of hearing too.

d. Anne wanted to be a teacher.

## 4. Helen Keller learned to speak but Anne translated her words when she spoke in public. The reason Helen needed a translator was because

a. Helen spoke another language.

b. Helen's words were hard for people to understand.

c. Helen spoke very quietly.

d. Helen did not speak but only used sign language.

**Questions 5 – 8 refer to the following passage.**

**Passage 2 - Ways Characters Communicate in Theater**

Playwrights give their characters voices in a way that gives depth and added meaning to what happens on stage during their play. There are different types of speech in scripts that allow characters to talk with themselves, with other characters, and even with the audience.

It is very unique to theater that characters may talk "to themselves." When characters do this, the speech they give is called a soliloquy. Soliloquies are usually poetic, introspective, moving, and can tell audience members about the feelings, motivations, or suspicions of an individual character without that character having to reveal them to other characters on stage. "To be or not to be" is a famous soliloquy given by Hamlet as he considers difficult but important themes, such as life and death.

The most common type of communication in plays is when one character is speaking to another or a group of other characters. This is generally called dialogue, but can also be called monologue if one character speaks without being interrupted for a long time. It is not necessarily the most important type of communication, but it is the most common because the plot of the play cannot really progress without it.

Lastly, and most unique to theater (although it has been used somewhat in film) is when a character speaks directly to the audience. This is called an aside, and scripts usually specifically direct actors to do this. Asides are usually comical, an inside joke between the character and the audience, and very short. The actor will usually face the audience when delivering them, even if it's for a moment, so the audience can recognize this move as an aside.

All three of these types of communication are important to the art of theater, and have been perfected by famous playwrights like Shakespeare. Understanding these types of communication can help an audience member grasp what is artful about the script and action of a play.

**5. According to the passage, characters in plays communicate to**

    a. move the plot forward

    b. show the private thoughts and feelings of one character

    c. make the audience laugh

    d. add beauty and artistry to the play

**6. When Hamlet delivers "To be or not to be," he can be described as**

    a. solitary

    b. thoughtful

    c. dramatic

    d. hopeless

**7. The author uses parentheses to punctuate "although it has been used somewhat in film,"**

   a. to show that films are less important

   b. instead of using commas so that the sentence is not interrupted

   c. because parenthesis help separate details that are not as important

   d. to show that films are not as artistic

**Questions 9 – 11 refer to the following passage.**

**Passage 3 - Low Blood Sugar**

As the name suggest, low blood sugar is low sugar levels in the bloodstream. This can occur when you have not eaten properly and undertake strenuous activity, or, when you are very hungry. When Low blood sugar occurs regularly and is ongoing, it is a medical condition called hypoglycemia. This condition can occur in diabetics and in healthy adults.

Causes of low blood sugar can include excessive alcohol consumption, metabolic problems, stomach surgery, pancreas, liver or kidneys problems, as well as a side-effect of some medications.

**Symptoms**

There are different symptoms depending on the severity of the case.

Mild hypoglycemia can lead to feelings of nausea and hunger. The patient may also feel nervous, jittery and have fast heart beats. Sweaty skin, clammy and cold skin are likely symptoms.
Moderate hypoglycemia can result in a short temper, confusion, nervousness, fear and blurring of vision. The patient may feel weak and unsteady.

Severe cases of hypoglycemia can lead to seizures, coma, fainting spells, nightmares, headaches, excessive sweats and severe tiredness.

## Diagnosis of low blood sugar

A doctor can diagnosis this medical condition by asking the patient questions and testing blood and urine samples. Home testing kits are available for patients to monitor blood sugar levels.  It is important to see a qualified doctor though.  The doctor can administer tests to ensure that will safely rule out other medical conditions that could affect blood sugar levels.

## Treatment

Quick treatments include drinking or eating foods and drinks with high sugar contents. Good examples include soda, fruit juice, hard candy and raisins. Glucose energy tablets can also help. Doctors may also recommend medications and well as changes in diet and exercise routine to treat chronic low blood sugar.

**8. Based on the article, which of the following is true?**

    a. Low blood sugar can happen to anyone.

    b. Low blood sugar only happens to diabetics.

    c.  Low blood sugar can occur even.

    d. None of the statements are true.

**9. Which of the following are the author's opinion?**

    a. Quick treatments include drinking or eating foods and drinks with high sugar contents.

    b. None of the statements are opinions.

    c.  This condition can occur in diabetics and in healthy adults.

    d. There are different symptoms depending on the severity of the case

### 10. What is the author's purpose?

    a. To inform

    b. To persuade

    c. To entertain

    d. To analyze

### 11. Which of the following is not a detail?

    a. A doctor can diagnosis this medical condition by asking the patient questions and testing.

    b. A doctor will test blood and urine samples.

    c. Glucose energy tablets can also help.

    d. Home test kits monitor blood sugar levels.

### Questions 12 – 15 refer to the following passage.

### How To Get A Good Nights Sleep

Sleep is just as essential for healthy living as water, air and food. Sleep allows the body to rest and replenish depleted energy levels. Sometimes we may for various reasons experience difficulty sleeping which has a serious effect on our health. Those who have prolonged sleeping problems are facing a serious medical condition and should see a qualified doctor when possible for help. Here is simple guide that can help you sleep better at night.

Try to create a natural pattern of waking up and sleeping around the same time everyday. This means avoiding going to bed too early and oversleeping past your usual wake up time. Going to bed and getting up at radically different times everyday confuses your body clock. Try to establish a natural rhythm as much as you can.

Exercises and a bit of physical activity can help you sleep better at night. If you are having problem sleeping, try to be as active as you can during the day. If you are tired from physical activity, falling asleep is a natural and easy process for your body. If you remain inactive during the day, you will find it harder to sleep properly at night. Try walking, jogging, swimming or simple stretches as you get close to your bed time.

Afternoon naps are great to refresh you during the day, but they may also keep you awake at night. If you feel sleepy during the day, get up, take a walk and get busy to keep from sleeping. Stretching is a good way to increase blood flow to the brain and keep you alert so that you don't sleep during the day. This will help you sleep better night.

> A warm bath or a glass of milk in the evening
> can help your body relax and prepare for sleep. A cold bath will wake you up and keep
> you up for several hours. Also avoid eating too
> late before bed.

**12. How would you describe this sentence?**

   a. A recommendation

   b. An opinion

   c. A fact

   d. A diagnosis

**13. Which of the following is an alternative title for this article?**

   a. Exercise and a good night's sleep

   b. Benefits of a good night's sleep

   c. Tips for a good night's sleep

   d. Lack of sleep is a serious medical condition

**14. Which of the following cannot be inferred from this article?**

a. Biking is helpful for getting a good night's sleep

b. Mental activity is helpful for getting a good night's sleep

c. Eating bedtime snacks is not recommended

d. Getting up at the same time is helpful for a good night's sleep

**15. What is a disadvantage of taking naps?**

a. They may keep you awake.

b. There are no disadvantages

c. They may help you sleep better

d. They may affect your diet

**Question 16 refers to the following Table of Contents.**

**Contents**

**16. Consider the table of contents above. What page would you find information about natural selection and adaptation?**

    a. 81

    b. 90

    c. 110

    d. 132

**Questions 17 – 19 refer to the following passage.**

**Passage 5 - Pearl Harbor**

A Day That Will Live in Infamy! Attack on Pearl Harbor In 1941, the world was at war. The United States was trying to stay out of the conflict. In Europe, the countries of Germany and Italy had formed an alliance to expand their land and territory. Germany had already taken over Poland, Denmark, and parts of France. They were heading next toward England and due to all the fighting in Europe, there were battles taking place as far south as North Africa, where the German and Italian armies were fighting the British.

This got even worse when the Asian nation of Japan formed an alliance with Germany and Italy. Together, the three countries called themselves, the AXIS. Now, the war was in the Pacific as well as in Europe and Northern Africa. Many Americans felt that perhaps now was the time for the United States to join with its ally, Great Britain and stop the Axis from taking over more regions of the world.

In 1941, Franklin Roosevelt was President of the United States. His fear at the time was that Japan would try to take over many countries in Asia. He did not want to see that happen, so he moved some of the United States warships that had been stationed in San Diego, to the military base at Pearl Harbor, in Honolulu, Hawaii.

Japan quietly plotted their attack. They waited until the early hours of the morning on Sunday, December 7, 1941. Then, 350 Japanese war plans began to drop bombs on the U.S. ships at Pearl Harbor. The first bombs fell at 7:48

am and a mere 90 minutes later, the attack was over. Pearl Harbor was decimated. 8 battleships were damaged. Eleven ships were sunk and 300 U.S. planes were destroyed. Most devastating was the loss of life 2,400 U.S. military members was killed in the attack and 1, 282 were injured.

President Roosevelt addressed the country via the radio and said "Today is a day that will live in infamy." He asked Congress to declare war on Japan. War was declared on Japan on December 8th and on Germany and Italy on December 11th. The United States had entered World War Two.

**17. After reading the passage, we can infer infamy means?**

    a. Famous

    b. Remembered in a good way

    c. Remembered in a bad way

    d. Easily forgotten

**18. What three countries formed the Axis?**

    a. Italy, England, Germany

    b. United States, England, Italy

    c. Germany, Japan, Italy

    d. Germany, Japan, United States

**19. What do you think was President Roosevelt's reason for moving warships to Pearl Harbor?**

    a. He feared Japan would bomb San Diego

    b. He knew Japan was going to attack Pearl Harbor

    c. He was planning to attack Japan

    d. He wanted to try to protect Asian countries from Japanese takeover

**20. Why do you think Japan chose a Sunday morning at 7:48 am for their attack?**

    a. They knew the military slept late

    b. There is a law against bombing countries on a Sunday

    c. They wanted the attack to catch people by surprise

    d. That was the only free time they had to attack.

**Questions 21 - 24 refer to the following recipe.**

**If You Have Allergies, You're Not Alone**

People who experience allergies might joke that their immune systems have let them down or are seriously lacking. Truthfully though, people who experience allergic reactions or allergy symptoms during certain times of the year have heightened immune systems that are, "better" than those of people who have perfectly healthy but less militant immune systems.

Still, when a person has an allergic reaction, they are having an adverse reaction to a substance that is considered normal to most people. Mild allergic reactions usually have symptoms like itching, runny nose, red eyes, or bumps or discoloration of the skin. More serious allergic reactions, such as those to animal and insect poisons or certain foods, may result in the closing of the throat, swelling of the eyes, low blood pressure, inability to breath, and can even be fatal.

Different treatments help different allergies, and which one a person uses depends on the nature and severity of the allergy. It is recommended to patients with severe allergies to take extra precautions, such as carrying an EpiPen, which treats anaphylactic shock and may prevent death, always in order for the remedy to be readily available and more effective. When an allergy is not so severe, treatments may be used just relieve a person of uncomfortable symptoms. Over the counter allergy medicines treat milder symptoms, and can be bought at any grocery store and used in moderation to help people with allergies live normally.

There are many tests available to assess whether a person has allergies or what they may be allergic to, and advances in these tests and the medicine used to treat patients continues to improve. Despite this fact, allergies still affect many people throughout the year or even every day. Medicines used to treat allergies have side-effects, and it is difficult to bring the body into balance with the use of medicine. Regardless, many of those who live with allergies are grateful for what is available and find it useful in maintaining their lifestyles.

**21. According to this passage, which group does the word "militant" belong in**

    a. sickly, ailing, faint

    b. strength, power, vigor

    c. active, fighting, warring

    d. worn, tired, breaking down

**22. The author says that "medicines used to treat allergies have side-effects of their own" to**

    a. point out that doctors aren't very good at diagnosing and treating allergies

    b. argue that because of the large number of people with allergies, a cure will never be found

    c. explain that allergy medicines aren't cures and some compromise must be made

    d. argue that more wholesome remedies should be researched and medicines banned

**23. It can be inferred that _____ recommend that some people with allergies carry medicine with them.**

   a. the author

   b. doctors

   c. the makers of EpiPen

   d. people with allergies

**24. The author has written this passage to**

   a. inform readers on symptoms of allergies so people with allergies can get help

   b. persuade readers to be proud of having allergies

   c. inform readers on different remedies so people with allergies receive the right help

   d. describe different types of allergies, their symptoms, and their remedies

**Questions 25 – 26 refer to the following email.**

SUBJECT:  MEDICAL STAFF CHANGES

To all staff:

This email is to advise you of a paper on recommended medical staff changes has been posted to the Human Resources website.

The contents are of primary interest to medical staff, other staff may be interested in reading it, particularly those in medical support roles.

The paper deals with several major issues:

   1. Improving our ability to attract top quality staff to the hospital, and retain our existing staff.  These changes will make our position and departmental names internationally recognizable and comparable with North American and North Asian departments and positions.

2. Improving our ability to attract top quality staff by introducing greater flexibility in the departmental structure.

3. General comments on issues to be further discussed relative to research staff.

The changes outlined in this paper are significant. I encourage you to read the document and send to me any comments you may have, so that it can be enhanced and improved.

Gordon Simms
Administrator,
Seven Oaks Regional Hospital

**25. Are all hospital staff required to read the document posted to the Human Resources website?**

    a. Yes all staff are required to read the document.

    b. No, reading the document is optional.

    c. Only medical staff are required to read the document.

    d. none of the above are correct.

**26. Have the changes to medical staff been made?**

    a. Yes, the changes have been made.

    b. No, the changes are only being discussed.

    c. Some of the changes have been made.

    d. None of the choices are correct.

**Questions 27 – 30 refer to the following passage.**

**When a Poet Longs to Mourn, He Writes an Elegy**

Poems are an expressive, especially emotional, form of writing. They have been in literature virtually from the time civilizations invented the written word. Poets often portrayed as moody, secluded, and even troubled, but this is because poets are introspective and feel deeply about the current events and cultural norms they are surrounded with. Poets often produce the most telling literature, giving insight into the society and mind-set they come from. This can be done in many forms.

The oldest types of poems often include many stanzas, may or may not rhyme, and are more about telling a story than experimenting with language or words. The most common types of ancient poetry are epics, which are usually extremely long stories that follow a hero through his journey, or ellegies, which are often solemn in tone and used to mourn or lament something or someone. The Mesopotamians are often said to have invented the written word, and their literature is among the oldest in the world, including the epic poem titled "Epic of Gilgamesh." Similar in style and length to "Gilgamesh" is "Beowulf," an ellegy written in Old English and set in Scandinavia. These poems are often used by professors as the earliest examples of literature.

The importance of poetry was revived in the Renaissance. At this time, Europeans discovered the style and beauty of ancient Greek arts, and poetry was among those. Shakespeare is the most well-known poet of the time, and he used poetry not only to write poems but also to write plays for the theater. The most popular forms of poetry during the Renaissance included villanelles, (a nineteen-line poetic form) sonnets, as well as the epic. Poets during this time focused on style and form, and developed very specific rules and outlines for how an exceptional poem should be written.

As often happens in the arts, modern poets have rejected the constricting rules of Renaissance poets, and free form poems are much more popular. Some modern poems would read just like stories if they weren't arranged into lines and stanzas. It is difficult to tell which poems and poets will be the most important, because works of art often become more famous in hindsight, after the poet has died and society can look at itself without being in the moment. Modern poetry continues to develop, and will no doubt continue to change as values, thought, and writing continue to change.

Poems can be among the most enlightening and uplifting texts for a person to read if they are looking to connect with the past, connect with other people, or try to gain an understanding of what is happening in their time.

**27. In summary, the author has written this passage**

   a. as a foreword that will introduce a poem in a book or magazine

   b. because she loves poetry and wants more people to like it

   c. to give a brief history of poems

   d. to convince students to write poems

**28. The author organizes the paragraphs mainly by**

   a. moving chronologically, explaining which types of poetry were common in that time

   b. talking about new types of poems each paragraph and explaining them a little

   c. focusing on one poet or group of people and the poems they wrote

   d. explaining older types of poetry so she can talk about modern poetry

**29. The author's claim that poetry has been around "virtually from the time civilizations invented the written word" is supported by the detail that**

   a. Beowulf is written in Old English, which is not really in use any longer

   b. epic poems told stories about heroes

   c. the Renaissance poets tried to copy Greek poets

   d. the Mesopotamians are credited with both inventing the word and writing "Epic of Gilgamesh"

**30. According to the passage, the word "telling" means**

    a. speaking

    b. significant

    c. soothing

    d. wordy

**Questions 31 – 32 refer to the following passage.**

**Scottish Wind Farms**

The Scottish Government has a targeted plan of generating 100% of Scotland's electricity through renewable energy by 2020. Renewable energy sources include sun, water and wind power. Scotland uses all forms but its fastest growing energy is wind energy. Wind power is generated by wind turbines, placed onshore and offshore. Wind turbines that are grouped together in large numbers are called wind farms. A majority of Scottish citizens say that the wind farms are necessary to meet current and future energy needs, and would like to see an increase in the number of wind farms.  They cite the fact that wind energy does not cause pollution, there are low operational costs, and most importantly, by definition, renewable energy it cannot be depleted.

**31. What is Scotland's fastest growing source of renewable energy?**

    a. Solar Panels

    b. Hydroelectric

    c. Wind

    d. Fossil Fuels

**32. Why do the majority of Scottish citizens agree with the Government's plan?**

    a. Their concern for current and future energy needs

    b. Because of the low operational costs

    c. Because they are out of sight

    d. Because it provides jobs

**Questions 33 – 35 refer to the following passage.**

**Scottish Wind Farms II**

However, there is still a public debate concerning the use of wind farms to generate energy. The most cited argument against wind energy is that the upfront investment is expensive. They also argue that it is aesthetically displeasing, they are noisy, and they create a serious threat to wildlife in the area. While wind energy is renewable, or cannot be depleted, it does not mean that wind is always available. Wind is fluctuating, or intermittent, and therefore not suited to meet the base energy demand, meaning if there is no wind then no energy is being created.

**33. What is the biggest argument against wind energy?**

    a. The turbines are noisy

    b. The turbines endanger wildlife

    c. The turbines are expensive to build

    d. They are aesthetically displeasing

**34. What is the best way to describe this article's description of wind energy?**

    a. Loud and ever present

    b. The cheapest form of renewable energy

    c. The only source of renewable energy in Scotland

    d. Clean and renewable but fluctuating

Save the Children

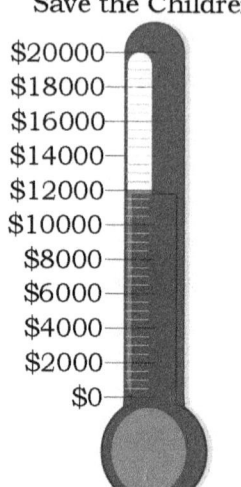

**35. Consider the graphic above. The Save the Children fund has a fund-raising goal of $20,000. Approximately how much of their goal have they achieved?**

    a. 3/5

    b. 3/4

    c. 1/2

    d. 1/3

# Section II – Math

### 1. What is 1/3 of 3/4?

    a.  1/4

    b.  1/3

    c.  2/3

    d.  3/4

### 2. What fraction of $1500 is $75?

    a. 1/14

    b. 3/5

    c. 7/10

    d. 1/20

### 3. 3.14 + 2.73 + 23.7 =

    a.  28.57

    b.  30.57

    c.  29.56

    d.  29.57

### 4. A woman spent 15% of her income on an item and ends with $120. What percentage of her income is left?

    a.  12%

    b.  85%

    c.  75%

    d.  95%

### 5. Express 0.27 + 0.33 as a fraction.

    a.  3/6

    b.  4/7

    c.  3/5

    d.  2/7

**6. What is (3.13 + 7.87) X 5?**

    a. 65

    b. 50

    c. 45

    d. 55

**7. Reduce 2/4 X 3/4 to lowest terms.**

    a. 6/12

    b. 3/8

    c. 6/16

    d. 3/4

**8. 2/3 – 2/5 =**

    a. 4/10

    b. 1/15

    c. 3/7

    d. 4/15

**9. 2/7 + 2/3 =**

    a. 12/23

    b. 5/10

    c. 20/21

    d. 6/21

**10. 2/3 of 60 + 1/5 of 75 =**

    a. 45

    b. 55

    c. 15

    d. 50

**11. 8 is what percent of 40?**

    a. 10%

    b. 15%

    c. 20%

    d. 25%

**12. 9 is what percent of 36?**

    a. 10%

    b. 15%

    c. 20%

    d. 25%

**13. Three tenths of 90 equals:**

    a. 18

    b. 45

    c. 27

    d. 36

**14. .4% of 36 is**

    a. 1.44

    b. .144

    c. 14.4

    d. 144

15. The physician ordered 5 mg Coumadin; 10 mg/tablet is on hand. How many tablets will you give?

    a.  .5 tablets

    b.  1 tablet

    c.  .75 tablets

    d.  1.5 tablets

16. The physician ordered 20 mg Tylenol/kg of body weight; on hand is 80 mg/tablet. The child weighs 12 kg. How many tablets will you give?

    a.  1 tablet

    b.  3 tablets

    c.  2 tablets

    d.  4 tablets

17. The physician ordered 20 mg Tylenol/kg of body weight; on hand is 80 mg/tablet. The child weighs 44 lb. How many tablets will you give?

    a.  5 tablets

    b.  5.5 tablets

    c.  4.5 tablets

    d.  3 tablets

18. The physician ordered 3,000 units of heparin; 5,000 U/mL is on hand. How many milliliters will you give?

    a.  0.5 ml

    b.  0.6 ml

    c.  0.75 ml

    d.  0.8 ml

19. The physician orders 60 mg Augmentin; 80 mg/mL is on hand. How many milliliters will you give?

    a.  1 ml

    b.  0.5 ml

    c.  0.75 ml

    d.  0.95 ml

20. The physician ordered 16 mg Ibuprofen/kg of body weight; on hand is 80 mg/tablet. The child weighs 15 kg. How many tablets will you give?

    a.  3 tablets

    b.  2 tablets

    c.  1 tablet

    d.  2.5 tablets

**21. The physician orders 1000 mg Benbadryl liquid; 1 g/tsp is on hand. How many teaspoons will you give?**

    a.  .75 tsp

    b.  1.5 tsp

    c.  1 tsp

    d.  1.25 tsp

**22. The physician ordered 10 units of regular insulin and 200 U/mL is on hand. How many milliliters will you give?**

    a.  .45 ml

    b.  .75 ml

    c.  .25 ml

    d.  .05 ml

**23. If y = 4 and x = 3, solve $yx^3$**

    a.  -108

    b.  108

    c.  27

    d.  4

**24. Convert 0.007 kilograms to grams**

    a.  7 grams

    b.  70 grams

    c.  0.07 grams

    d.  0.70 grams

**25. Convert 16 quarts to gallons**

    a.  1 gallons

    b.  8 gallons

    c.  4 gallons

    d.  4.5 gallons

**26. Convert 2 teaspoons to milliliters.**

    a.  4.3 milliliters

    b.  9 milliliters

    c.  9.86 milliliters

    d.  4 milliliters

**27. Convert 200 meters to kilometers**

    a.  50 kilometers

    b.  20 kilometers

    c.  12 kilometers

    d.  0.2 kilometers

**28. Convert 72 inches to feet**

    a.  12 feet

    b.  6 feet

    c.  4 feet

    d.  17 feet

**29. Convert 3 yards to feet**

    a.  18 feet

    b.  12 feet

    c.  9 feet

    d.  27 feet

**30. Convert 45 kg. to pounds.**

   a. 10 pounds

   b. 100 pounds

   c. 1,000 pounds

   d. 110 pounds

**31. Convert 0.63 grams to mg.**

   a. 630 g.

   b. 63 mg.

   c. 630 mg.

   d. 603 mg.

**32. $5x + 3 = 7x -1$. Find x**

   a. 1/3

   b. ½

   c. 1

   d. 2

**33. $5x + 2(x + 7) = 14x - 7$. Find x**

   a. 1

   b. 2

   c. 3

   d. 4

**34. $12t -10 = 14t + 2$. Find t**

   a. -6

   b. -4

   c. 4

   d. 6

**35. $5(z + 1) = 3(z + 2) + 11$. Z =?**

   a. 2

   b. 4

   c. 6

   d. 12

**36. The price of a book went up from \$20 to \$25. What percent did the price increase?**

   a. 5%

   b. 10%

   c. 20%

   d. 25%

**37. The price of a book decreased from \$25 to \$20. What percent did the price decrease?**

   a. 5%

   b. 10%

   c. 20%

   d. 25%

**38. After taking several practice tests, Brian improved the results of his GRE test by 30%. Given that the first time he took the test Brian answered 150 questions correctly, how many questions did he answer correctly on the second test?**

   a. 105

   b. 120

   c. 180

   d. 195

**39.** In local baseball team, 4 players (or 12.5% of the team) have long hair and the rest have short hair. How many short-haired players are there on the team?

    a. 24

    b. 28

    c. 32

    d. 50

**40.** In the time required to serve 43 customers, a server breaks 2 glasses and slips 5 times. The next day, the same server breaks 10 glasses. Assuming the number of glasses broken is proportional to the number of customers served, how many customers did she serve?

    a. 25

    b. 43

    c. 86

    d. 215

**41.** A square lawn has an area of 62,500 square meters. What is the cost of building fence around it at a rate of $5.5 per meter?

    a. $4000

    b. $4500

    c. $5000

    d. $5500

**42.** Mr. Brown bought 5 cheese burgers, 3 drinks, and 4 fries for his family, and a cookie pack for his dog. If the price of all single items is the same at $1.30 and a 3.5% tax is added, what is the total cost of dinner for Mr. Brown?

    a. $16

    b. $16.9

    c. $17

    d. $17.5

**43.** The length of a rectangle is twice of its width and its area is equal to the area of a square with 12 cm. sides. What will be the perimeter of the rectangle to the nearest whole number?

    a. 36 cm

    b. 46 cm

    c. 51 cm

    d. 56 cm

**44.** There are 15 yellow and 35 orange balls in a basket. How many more yellow balls must be added to make the yellow balls 65%?

    a. 35

    b. 50

    c. 65

    d. 70

**45. A farmer wants to plant 65,536 trees in such a way that number of rows must be equal to the number of plants in a row. How many trees should he plant in a row?**

    a. 1684

    b. 1268

    c. 668

    d. 256

**46. A distributor purchased 550 kilograms of potatoes for $165. He distributed these at a rate of $6.4 per 20 kilograms to 15 shops, $3.4 per 10 kilograms to 12 shops and the remainder at $1.8 per 5 kilograms. If his total distribution cost is $10, what will his profit be?**

    a. $8.60

    b. $24.60

    c. $14.90

    d. $23.40

**47. A farmer wants to plant trees around the outside boundaries of his rectangular field of dimensions 650 meters × 780 meters. Each tree requires 5 meters of free space all around it from the stem. How many trees can he plant?**

    a. 572

    b. 568

    c. 286

    d. 282

**48. 3 boys are asked to clean a surface that is 4 ft². If the surface is divided equally among the boys, how much will each clean?**

    a. 1 ft 6 in²

    b. 14 in²

    c. 1 ft² in²

    d. 1 ft² 48 in²

**49. How much pay does Mr. Johnson receive if he gives half of his pay to his family, $250 to his landlord, and has exactly 3/7 of his pay left over?**

    a. $3600

    b. $3500

    c. $2800

    d. $1750

**50. A boy has 4 red, 5 green and 2 yellow balls. He chooses two balls randomly. What is the probability that one is red and other is green?**

    a.   2/11

    b.   19/22

    c.   20/121

    d.   9/11

# Section III – English Grammar

**1. Choose the sentence with the correct grammar.**

    a.   Don would never have thought of that book, but you could have reminded him.

    b.   Don would never of thought of that book, but you could have reminded him.

    c.   Don would never have thought of that book, but you could of have reminded him.

    d.   Don would never of thought of that book, but you could of reminded him.

**2. Choose the sentence with the correct grammar.**

    a. The man was asked to come with his daughter and her test results.

    b. The man was asked to come with her daughter and her test results.

    c. The man was asked to come with her daughter and our test results.

    d. None of the above.

**3. Choose the sentence with the proper usage.**

    a. They wanted to know if they may begin.

    b. They wanted to know if they might begin.

    c. None of the above.

**4. Choose the sentence with the correct grammar.**

a.  Although you may not see nobody in the dark, it does not mean that nobody is there.

b.  Although you may not see anyone in the dark, it does not mean that not nobody is there.

c.  Although you may not see anyone in the dark, it does not mean that no one is there.

d.  Although you may not see nobody in the dark, it does not mean that not nobody is there.

**5. Choose the sentence with the correct grammar.**

a. Any girl that fails the test loses their admission.

b. Any girl that fails the test loses our admission.

c. Any girl that fails the test loses her admission.

d. None of the above.

**6. Choose the sentence with the correct grammar.**

a.  The older children have already eat their dinner, but the baby has not yet eaten anything.

b.  The older children have already eaten their dinner, but the baby has not yet ate anything.

c.  The older children have already eaten their dinner, but the baby has not yet eaten anything.

d.  The older children have already eat their dinner, but the baby has not yet ate anything.

**7. Choose the sentence with the correct grammar.**

a.  If they had gone to the party, he would have gone, too.

b.  If they had went to the party, he would have gone, too.

c.  If they had gone to the party, he would have went, too.

d.  If they had went to the party, he would have went, too.

**8. Choose the sentence with the proper usage.**

    a. He can be correct.

    b. He could be correct.

    c. He may be correct.

    d. None of the above.

**9. Choose the sentence with the correct grammar.**

    a. Everyone was asked to raise their hand.

    b. Everyone was asked to raise our hand.

    c. Everyone was asked to raise her hand.

    d. None of the above.

**10. Choose the sentence with the correct grammar.**

    a. Its important for you to know its official name; its called the Confederate Museum.

    b. It's important for you to know it's official name; it's called the Confederate Museum.

    c. It's important for you to know its official name; it's called the Confederate Museum.

    d. Its important for you to know it's official name; it's called the Confederate Museum.

**11. The Ford Motor Company was named for Henry Ford, _____.**

    a. which had founded the company.

    b. who founded the company.

    c. whose had founded the company.

    d. whom had founded the company.

**12. Thomas Edison _____ since he invented the light bulb, television, motion pictures, and phonograph.**

 a. has always been known as the greatest inventor

 b. was always been known as the greatest inventor

 c. must have had been always known as the greatest inventor

 d. will had been known as the greatest inventor

**13. Choose the sentence with the proper usage.**

 a. I will be at the office by 9 a. m.

 b. I shall be at the office by 9 a. m.

 c. Both of the above

 d. None of the above

**14. Although Joe is tall for his age, his brother Elliot is _____ of the two.**

 a. the tallest

 b. more tallest

 c. the tall

 d. the taller

**15. When KISS came to town, all the tickets _____ before I could buy one.**

 a. will be sold out

 b. had been sold out

 c. were being sold out

 d. was sold out

**16. The rules of most sports _____ more complicated than we often realize.**

    a. are

    b. is

    c. was

    d. has been

**17. Choose the sentence with the correct grammar.**

    a. Here are the names of people whom you should contact

    b. Here are the names of people who you should contact

    c. Both of the above

    d. None of the above.

**18. The Titanic _____ mere days into its maiden voyage.**

    a. has already sunk

    b. will already sunk

    c. already sank

    d. sank

**19. _____ won first place in the Western Division?**

    a. Who

    b. Whom

    c. Which

    d. What

**20. There are now several ways to listen to music, including radio, CDs, and Mp3 files _____ you can download onto an MP3 player.**

    a. on which

    b. who

    c. whom

    d. which

**21. As the tallest monument in the United States, the St. Louis Arch _____.**

    a.  has rose to an impressive 630 feet.

    b.  is risen to an impressive 630 feet.

    c.  rises to an impressive 630 feet.

    d.  was rose to an impressive 630 feet.

**22. The tired, old woman should _____ on the sofa.**

    a.  lie

    b.  lays

    c.  laid

    d.  lain

**23. Did the students understand that Thanksgiving always _____ on the fourth Thursday in November?**

    a.  fallen

    b.  falling

    c.  has fell

    d.  falls

**24. Collecting stamps, _____ and listening to short-wave radio were Rick's main hobbies.**

    a.  building models,

    b.  to build models,

    c.  having built models,

    d.  build models,

**25. Choose the sentence with the correct usage.**

    a.  The ceremony had an emotional effect on the groom, but the bride was not affected.

    b.  The ceremony had an emotional affect on the groom, but the bride was not affected.

    c.  The ceremony had an emotional effect on the groom, but the bride was not effected.

    d.  The ceremony had an emotional affect on the groom, but the bride was not affected.

**26. Choose the sentence with the correct usage.**

a. Anna was taller then Luis, but then he grew four inches in three months.

b. Anna was taller then Luis, but than he grew four inches in three months.

c. Anna was taller than Luis, but than he grew four inches in three months.

d. Anna was taller than Luis, but then he grew four inches in three months.

**27. Choose the sentence with the correct usage.**

a. Their second home is in Boca Raton, but there not their for most of the year.

b. They're second home is in Boca Raton, but they're not there for most of the year.

c. Their second home is in Boca Raton, but they're not there for most of the year.

d. There second home is in Boca Raton, but they're not there for most of the year.

**28. Choose the sentence with the proper usage.**

a. He ought to be back by now.

b. He ought be back by now.

c. He ought come back by now.

d. None of the above.

**29. Choose the sentence with the correct grammar.**

a. Mark and Peter have talked to each other.

b. Mark and Peter have talked to one another.

c. Both of the above.

d. None of the above.

## 30. Choose the sentence with the correct usage.

a. You're classes are on the west side of campus, but you're living on the east side.

b. Your classes are on the west side of campus, but your living on the east side.

c. Your classes are on the west side of campus, but you're living on the east side.

d. You're classes are on the west side of campus, but you're living on the east side.

## 31. Choose the sentence with the correct usage.

a. Disease is highly prevalent in poorer nations; the most dominant disease is malaria.

b. Diseases are highly prevalent in poorer nations; the most dominant disease is malaria.

c. Disease is highly prevalent in poorer nations; the most dominant Diseases are malaria.

d. Diseases are highly prevalent in poorer nations; the most dominant Diseases are malaria.

## 32. Choose the sentence with the correct usage.

a. Although I would prefer to have dog, I actually own a cat.

b. Although I would prefer to have a dog, I actually own cat.

c. Although I would prefer to have a dog, I actually own a cat.

d. Although I would prefer to have dog, I actually own cat.

**33. Choose the sentence with the correct usage.**

a.  The principal of the school lived by one principle: always do your best.

b.  The principle of the school lived by one principle: always do your best.

c.  The principal of the school lived by one principal: always do your best.

d.  The principle of the school lived by one principal: always do your best.

**34. Choose the sentence with the correct usage.**

a.  Even with an speed limit sign clearly posted, an inattentive driver may drive too fast.

b.  Even with a speed limit sign clearly posted, a inattentive driver may drive too fast.

c.  Even with an speed limit sign clearly posted, a inattentive driver may drive too fast.

d.  Even with a speed limit sign clearly posted, an inattentive driver may drive too fast.

**35. Choose the sentence with the correct usage.**

a.  Except for the roses, she did not accept John's frequent gifts.

b.  Accept for the roses, she did not except John's frequent gifts.

c.  Accept for the roses, she did not accept John's frequent gifts.

d.  Except for the roses, she did not except John's frequent gifts.

## 36. Choose the sentence with the correct usage.

a. Although he continued to advise me, I no longer took his advice.

b. Although he continued to advice me, I no longer took his advise.

c. Although he continued to advise me, I no longer took his advise.

d. Although he continued to advice me, I no longer took his advise.

## 37. Choose the sentence with the correct usage.

a. To adopt to the climate, we had to adopt a different style of clothing.

b. To adapt to the climate, we had to adapt a different style of clothing.

c. To adapt to the climate, we had to adopt a different style of clothing.

d. To adapt to the climate, we had to adapt a different style of clothing.

## 38. Choose the sentence with the correct usage.

a. When he's between friends, Robert seems confident, but between you and me, he is really very shy.

b. When he's among friends, Robert seems confident, but among you and me, he is really very shy.

c. When he's between friends, Robert seems confident, but among you and me, he is really very shy.

d. When he's among friends, Robert seems confident, but between you and me, he is really very shy.

**39. Choose the sentence with the correct usage.**

a. I will be finished at ten in the morning, and will be arriving at home at about 6:30.

b. I will be finished at about ten in the morning, and will be arriving at home at 6:30.

c. I will be finished at about ten in the morning, and will be arriving at home at about 6:30.

d. I will be finished at ten in the morning, and will be arriving at home at 6:30.

**40. Choose the sentence with the correct usage.**

a. Beside the red curtains and pillows, there was a red rug beside the couch.

b. Besides the red curtains and pillows, there was a red rug beside the couch.

c. Besides the red curtains and pillows, there was a red rug besides the couch.

d. Beside the red curtains and pillows, there was a red rug besides the couch.

**41. Choose the sentence with the correct usage.**

a. Although John can swim very well, the lifeguard may not allow him to swim in the pool.

b. Although John may swim very well, the lifeguard may not allow him to swim in the pool.

c. Although John can swim very well, the lifeguard cannot allow him to swim in the pool.

d. Although John may swim very well, the lifeguard may not allow him to swim in the pool.

**42. Choose the sentence with the correct usage.**

a. Her continuous absences caused a continual disruption at the office.

b. Her continual absences caused a continuous disruption at the office.

c. Her continual absences caused a continual disruption at the office.

d. Her continuous absences caused a continuous disruption at the office.

**43. Choose the sentence with the correct usage.**

a. During the famine, the Irish people had to emigrate to other countries; many of them immigrated to the United States.

b. During the famine, the Irish people had to immigrate to other countries; many of them immigrated to the United States.

c. During the famine, the Irish people had to emigrate to other countries; many of them emigrated to the United States.

d. During the famine, the Irish people had to immigrate to other countries; many of them emigrated to the United States.

**44. Choose the sentence with the correct usage.**

a. His home was farther than we expected; farther, the roads were very bad.

b. His home was farther than we expected; further, the roads were very bad.

c. His home was further than we expected; further, the roads were very bad.

d. His home was further than we expected; farther, the roads were very bad.

**45. Choose the sentence with the correct usage.**

a. The volunteers brought groceries and toys to the homeless shelter; the latter were given to the staff, while the former were given directly to the children.

b. The volunteers brought groceries and toys to the homeless shelter; the former was given to the staff, while the latter was given directly to the children.

c. The volunteers brought groceries and toys to the homeless shelter; the groceries were given to the staff, while the former was given directly to the children.

d. The volunteers brought groceries and toys to the homeless shelter; the latter was given to the staff, while the groceries were given directly to the children.

**46. Choose the sentence with the correct usage.**

a. Vegetables are a healthy food; eating them can make you more healthful.

b. Vegetables are a healthful food; eating them can make you more healthful.

c. Vegetables are a healthy food; eating them can make you more healthy.

d. Vegetables are a healthful food; eating them can make you more healthy.

**47. Choose the sentence with the correct usage.**

a. After you lay the books on the counter, you may lay down for a nap.

b. After you lie the books on the counter, you may lay down for a nap.

c. After you lay the books on the counter, you may lie down for a nap.

d. After you lay the books on the counter, you may lay down for a nap.

**48. Choose the sentence with the correct usage.**

a. After you lay the books on the counter, you may lay down for a nap.

b. After you lie the books on the counter, you may lay down for a nap.

c. After you lay the books on the counter, you may lie down for a nap.

d. After you lay the books on the counter, you may lay down for a nap.

**49. Choose the sentence with the correct usage.**

a. Once the chickens had layed their eggs, they lay on their nests to hatch them.

b. Once the chickens had lay their eggs, they lay on their nests to hatch them.

c. Once the chickens had laid their eggs, they lay on their nests to hatch them.

d. Once the chickens had laid their eggs, they laid on their nests to hatch them.

**50. Choose the sentence with the correct usage.**

a. Mrs. Foster taught me many things, but I learned the most from Mr. Wallace.

b. Mrs. Foster learned me many things, but I was taught the most by Mr. Wallace.

c. Mrs. Foster learned me many things, but I learned the most from Mr. Wallace.

d. Mrs. Foster taught me many things, but I was learned the most from Mr. Wallace.

# Section IV – Vocabulary

**1. Choose a verb that means fearless or invulnerable to intimidation and fear.**

    a. Feeble

    b. Strongest

    c. Dauntless

    d. Super

**2. Choose a word that means the same as the underlined word.**

**I see the differences when they are placed side-by-side and <u>juxtaposed</u>.**

    a. Compared

    b. Eliminated

    c. Overturned

    d. Exonerated

**3. Choose the best definition of regicide.**

    a. v. To endow or furnish with requisite ability, character, knowledge and skill

    b. n. killing of a king

    c. adj. Disposed to seize by violence or by unlawful or greedy methods

    d. v. To refresh after labor

**4. Choose the best definition of pernicious.**

    a. Deadly

    b. Infectious

    c. Common

    d. Rare

**5. Fill in the blank.**

**After she received her influenza vaccination, Nan thought that she was _____ to the common cold.**

    a. Immune

    b. Susceptible

    c. Vulnerable

    d. At risk

**6. Choose a word that means the same as the underlined word.**

**She performed the gymnastics and stretches so well! I have never seen anyone so <u>nimble</u>.**

    a. Awkward

    b. Agile

    c. Quick

    d. Taut

**7. Choose a word that means the same as the underlined word.**

**Are there any more <u>queries</u>? We have already had so many questions today.**

    a. Questions

    b. Commands

    c. Obfuscations

    d. Paradoxes

**8. Choose a verb that means to remove a leader or high official from position.**

    a. Sack

    b. Suspend

    c. Depose

    d. Dropped

**9. Choose the best definition of pedestrian.**

    a. Rare

    b. Often

    c. Walking or Running

    d. Commonplace

**10. Choose the best definition of petulant.**

    a. Patient

    b. Childish

    c. Impatient

    d. Mature

**11. Fill in the blank.**

**Paul's rose bushes were being destroyed by Japanese beetles, so he invested in a good _____.**

    a. Fungicide

    b. Fertilizer

    c. Sprinkler

    d. Pesticide

**12. Choose the best definition of salient.**

    a. v. To make light by fermentation, as dough

    b. adj. Not stringent or energetic

    c. adj. negligible

    d. adj. worthy of note or relevant

**13. Choose the best definition of sedentary.**

    a. n. A morbid condition, due to obstructed excretion of bile or characterized by yellowing of the skin

    b. adj. not moving or sitting at a place

    c. v. To wander from place to place

    d. n. Perplexity

**14. Fill in the blank.**

**The last time that the crops failed, the entire nation experienced months of _____.**

   a. Famine

   b. Harvest

   c. Plenitude

   d. Disease

**15. Choose the best definition of stint.**

   a. Thrifty

   b. Annoyed

   c. Dislike

   d. Insult

**16. Choose the best definition of precipitate.**

   a. To rain

   b. To throw down

   c. To throw up

   d. to snow

**17. Choose the verb that means to build up or strengthen relative to morals or religion.**

   a. Sanctify

   b. Amplify

   c. Edify

   d. Wry

**18. Choose the noun that means exit or way out.**

   a. Door-jamb

   b. Egress

   c. Regress

   d. Furtherance

**19. Choose the best definition of the underlined word.**

**The tide was in this morning but now it is starting to <u>recede</u>.**

a. Go out

b. Flow

c. Swell

d. Come in

**20. Choose the word that means private, personal.**

a. Confidential

b. Hysteric

c. Simplistic

d. Promissory

**21. Choose the best definition of the underlined word.**

**I don't think that will make it any better - it is just going to <u>aggravate</u> the situation.**

a. Worsen

b. Precipitate

c. Elongate

d. None of the above

**22. Choose the best definition of the underlined word.**

**I didn't think this was her first appearance, but it is her <u>debut</u>.**

a. Exit

b. Introduction

c. Curtain Call

d. Resignation

**23. Fill in the blank.**

**Because of a pituitary dysfunction, Karl lacked the necessary _____ to grow as tall as his father.**

    a. Glands
    b. Hormones
    c. Vitamins
    d. Testosterone

**24. Choose the best definition of importune.**

    a. To find an opportunity
    b. To ask all the time
    c. Cannot find an opportunity
    d. None of the above

**25. Choose the best definition of sedulous.**

    a. n. The support on or against which a lever rests
    b. adj. constant steady pursuit
    c. v. To oppose with an equal force
    d. n. The branch of medical science that relates to improving health

**26. Choose the best definition of tincture.**

    a. n. alcoholic drink with plant extract used for medicine
    b. n. An artificial trance-sleep
    c. n. a special medicinal drink made by mixing water with plant extracts
    d. adj. the point of puncture

**27. Choose the noun that means serious criminal offence that is punishable by death or imprisonment above a year**

a. Trespass

b. Hampers

c. Felony

d. Obligatory

**28. Choose the best meaning of the underlined word.**

**His library is enormous. I didn't realize he was such a bibliophile.**

a. Book lover

b. Audiophile

c. Bibliophobe

d. Audiophobe

**29. Fill in the blank.**

**When Mr. Davis returned from southern Asia, he told us about the _____ that sometimes swept the area, bringing torrential rain.**

a. Monsoons

b. Hurricanes

c. Blizzards

d. Floods

**30. Choose the best definition of volatile.**

a. Not explosive

b. Catches fire easily

c. Does not catch fire

d. Explosive

**31. Choose the word that means the same as plaintive.**

a. Happy

b. Mournful

c. Faint

d. Plain

**32. What is the best definition of truism?**

a. n. A comparison which directs the mind to the representative object itself

b. n. self-evident or clear obvious truth

c. n. a statement that is true but that can hardly be proved

d. n. false statements

**33. Choose the verb that means to encourage or incite troublesome acts.**

a. Comment

b. Foment

c. Integument

d. Atonement

**34. Choose the adjective that means dignified, solemn that is appropriate for a funeral.**

a. Funereal

b. Prediction

c. Wailing

d. Vociferous

**35. Choose the best definition for the underlined word.**

**I thought they were being very discreet, but they were, in fact, very <u>flagrant</u>.**

    a. Obvious

    b. Secretive

    c. Hidden

    d. Subtle

**36. Fill in the blank.**

**Is it true that _____ always grows on the north side of trees?**

    a. Lichens

    b. Moss

    c. Ferns

    d. Ground cover

**37. Choose the best definition of nexus.**

    a. A connection

    b. A telephone switch

    c. Part of a computer

    d. None of the above.

**38. Choose the best definition of zealot.**

    a. n. a person who is very passionate and fanatic about his specific objectives or beliefs

    b. n. The property or state of allowing the passage of light

    c. adj. Existing for a short time only

    d. n. An interpreter

## 39. Choose the best definition of vertigo.

   a.  n. Hard or agonizing labor

   b.  n. dizziness

   c.  n. a spicy shrub found on the mountain plains of East Africa

   d.  adj. pain caused by falling from a high height

## 40. Choose the best definition of trenchant.

   a. adj. Vigorous or incisive in expression or style.

   b. n. A specific capability of feeling or emotion

   c. n. A word having the same or almost the same meaning as some other

   d. n. a military jacket that is also bullet proof

## 41. Choose the noun that means warmth and kindness of disposition.

   a. Seethe

   b. Geniality

   c. Desists

   d. Predicate

## 42. He goes for coffee everyday.  It is his habitual start to the day.

   a.  Customary

   b. Rare

   c. Unchanging

   d. Unusual

**43. Choose the best definition for the underlined word.**

**She is just crazy about Britney Spears. She <u>idolizes</u> her a little too much I think.**

    a. Fears

    b. Worships

    c. Rejects

    d. Refutes

**44. Choose the best definition of osculate.**

    a. v. to rotate anti clockwise

    b. v. to rescue

    c. v. to kiss or related to kissing

    d. v. to break into little pieces

**45. Choose the best definition of conjoin.**

    a. A connection

    b. To marry

    c. Weld together

    d. To join together

**46. Choose the best definition of petrify.**

    a. Turn into a fossil

    b. Turn to stone

    c. Turn into wood

    d. Turn into glass

**47. Fill in the blank.**

**You can _____ some fires by covering them with dirt, while others require foam or water.**

    a. Extinguish

    b. Distinguish

    c. Ignite

    d. Lessen

**48. Fill in the blank.**

**Through powerful fans that circulate the heat over the food, _____ ovens work very efficiently.**

 a. Microwave

 b. Broiler

 c. Convection

 d. Pressure

**49. Select the word that means the same as the under-lined word.**

**She has been to some very dangerous places.  She is an <u>intrepid</u> explorer.**

 a. Brave

 b. Timid

 c. Timorous

 d. Cowardly

**50. Choose the verb that means to encourage, stimulate or incite and provoke.**

 a. Push

 b. Force

 c. Threaten

 d. Goad

# Section V – Science

**1. A motorcycle traveling 90 mph accelerates to pass a truck. Five seconds later the motorcycle is going 120 mph. Calculate the motorcycles' acceleration.**

    a.  6 mph/second$^2$

    b.  10 mph/second$^2$

    c.  15 mph/second$^2$

    d.  20 mph/second$^2$

**2. Which of the following disciplines have a close relationship with cell biology?**

    a.  Genetics

    b.  Genealogy

    c.  Paleontology

    d.  Archaeology

**3. A solution with a pH value of greater than 7 is**

    a. Base

    b. Acid

    c. Neutral

    d. None of the above

**4. Ohm's law states**

    a. The voltage across a resistor is not equal to the product of the resistance and the current flowing through it.

    b. The voltage across a resistor is equal to the product of the resistance and the current flowing through it.

    c. The voltage across a resistor is greater than the product of the resistance.

    d. The voltage across a resistor is equal to the current flowing through it.

## 5. Which statement below regarding Eukaryotic and prokaryotic cells is correct?

a. Both are organelles

b. Eukaryotic are not organelles

c. Both have DNA

d. Both have single membrane compartments

## 6. Electricity is a general term encompassing a variety of phenomena resulting from the presence and flow of electric charge. Which of the following statements about electricity is/are true?

a. Electrically charged matter is influenced by, and produces, electromagnetic fields.

b. Electric current is a movement or flow of electrically charged particles.

c. Electric potential is a fundamental interaction between the magnetic field and the presence and motion of an electric charge.

d. An influence produced by an electric charge on other charges in its vicinity is an electric field.

## 7. Which of these is not a process involved in cellular biology?

a. Active transport

b. Adhesion

c. Subversion

d. Cell signaling

## 8. When we say that important traits for scientific classification are homologous, "homologous" means

a. Being shared among two or more animals with the same parent.

b. Being coincidentally shared by two totally different creatures.

c. Being inherited by the organisms' common ancestors.

d. Mutating beyond all reasonable expectations.

**9. The manner in which instructions for building proteins, the basic structural molecules of living material are written in the DNA, is**

a. Genotypic assignment

b. Chromosome pattern

c. Genetic code

d. Genetic fingerprinting

**10. A _____ is a unit of inherited material, encoded by a strand of DNA and transcribed by RNA.**

a. Allele

b. Phenotype

c. Gene

d. Genotype

**11. A runner can sprint 6 meters per second. How far will she travel in 2 minutes?**

a. 600 meters

b. 720 meters

c. 760 meters

d. 800 meters

**12. Which of these is not an area studied in cell biology?**

a. Cells physiological properties

b. Cell structure

c. Cell life cycle

d. Cellular scientists' biographies

**13. Why is detection of pathogens complicated?**

a. They evolve so quickly

b. They die so quickly

c. They are invisible

d. They multiply so quickly

**14. Calculate the molarity of a sugar solution if 4 liters of the solution contains 8 moles of sugar?**

    a. 0.5 M

    b. 8 M

    c. 2 M

    d. 80 M

**15. Which of the following is/are not included in Ohm's Law?**

    a. Ohm's Law defines the relationships between (P) power, (E) voltage, (I) current, and (R) resistance.

    b. One ohm is the resistance value through which one volt will maintain a current of one ampere.

    c. Using Ohm's Law, voltage is determined using V = IR, with I equaling current and R equaling resistance.

    d. An ohm ($\Omega$) is a unit of electrical voltage.

**16. How many elements are represented on the modern periodic table?**

    a. 122 elements

    b. 99 elements

    c. 102 elements

    d. 118 elements

**17. Which, if any, of the following statements are false?**

    a. A mutation is a permanent change in the DNA sequence of a gene.

    b. Mutations in a gene's DNA sequence can alter the amino acid sequence of the protein encoded by the gene.

    c. Mutations in DNA sequences usually occur spontaneously.

    d. Mutations in DNA sequences can caused by exposure to environmental agents such as sunshine.

**18. Three cars are traveling down an even road at a velocity of 110 m/s, calculate the car with the highest momentum if they are all moving at the same speed, but the first car weighs 2500 kg, second car weighs 2650 kg and third car weighs 2009 kg?**

 a. First car

 b. Second car

 d. Third car

 d. All have same momentum

**19. Starting with the weakest, arrange the fundamental forces of nature in order of strength.**

 a. Gravity, Weak Nuclear Force, Electromagnetic Force, Strong Nuclear Force

 b. Weak Nuclear Force, Gravity, Electromagnetic Force, Strong Nuclear Force

 c. Strong Nuclear Force, Weak Nuclear Force, Electromagnetic Force, Gravity

 d. Gravity, Strong Nuclear Force, Weak Nuclear Force, Electromagnetic Force

**20. What are electrons?**

 a. Subatomic particles that carry a negative charge

 b. Subatomic particles that carry a positive charge

 c. Subatomic particles that carry both a negative and positive charge

 d. None of the above

**21. Cell culture is defined as**

 a. The technique for growing cells independent of a living organism within the confines of a laboratory.

 b. The process of killing cells through use of lasers.

 c. The method of creating cellular communities.

 d. A method for localizing proteins in tissue slices.

**22. _____, which refers to the repeatability of measurement, does not require knowledge of the correct or true value.**

    a. Precision

    b. Value

    c. Certainty

    d. Accuracy

**23. Describe a conductor.**

    a. A conductor contains a moving electrical charge.

    b. A conductor will move an electrical charge depending on the size.

    c. A conductor contains an electrical charge which will move when an electric potential difference is applied.

    d. None of the above

**24. Describe the periodic table.**

    a. The periodic table is a tabular display of the chemical compounds organized on the basis of their atomic numbers, electron configurations, and recurring chemical properties.

    b. The periodic table is a tabular display of the chemical elements, organized on the basis of their atomic numbers, electron configurations, and recurring chemical properties.

    c. The periodic table is a tabular display of the chemical subatomic particles, organized on the basis of their atomic numbers, electron configurations, and recurring chemical properties.

    d. None of the above.

**25. The scientific discipline that studies the physiological aspects, structures, life cycles and division of cells is called _____.**

    a. Physiology

    b. Cell science

    c. Biochemistry

    d. Cell biology

**26. What is the minimum amount of energy required to remove an electron from an atom or ion in the gas phase?**

    a. Ionization energy

    b. Valence energy

    c. Atomic energy

    d. Ionic energy

**27. In a redox reaction, the number of electrons lost is**

    a. Less than the number of electrons gained

    b. More than the number of electrons gained

    c. Equal to the number of electrons gained

    d. None of the above

**28.  In terms of the scientific method, the term _____ refers to the act of noticing or perceiving something and/or recording a fact or occurrence.**

    a. Observation

    b. Diligence

    c. Perception

    d. Control

**29. The _____ Theory defines acids and bases in terms of the electron-pair concept; according to its definition, an acid is an electron-pair acceptor, and a base is an electron-pair donor.**

   a. Arrhenius
   b. Lewis
   c. Clark
   d. Brønstead-Lowry

**30. What is the molarity of a solution containing 5 moles of solute in 250 milliliters of solution?**

   a. 20 M
   b. 15 M
   c. 0.104 M
   d. 1.25 M

**31. The property of a conductor that restricts its internal flow of electrons is:**

   a. Friction
   b. Power
   c. Current
   d. Resistance

**32. Describe bacteria.**

   a. Prokaryotic microorganisms that are usually just a few micrometers long.
   b. A single-celled organism.
   c. A virus.
   d. Three or more molecules clumped together.

**33. What is the difference, of any, between kinetic energy and potential energy?**

a. Kinetic energy is the energy of a body that results from heat while potential energy is the energy possessed by an object that is chilled.

b. Kinetic energy is the energy of a body that results from motion while potential energy is the energy possessed by an object by virtue of its position or state, e.g., as in a compressed spring.

c. There is no difference between kinetic and potential energy; all energy is the same.

d. Potential energy is the energy of a body that results from motion while kinetic energy is the energy possessed by an object by virtue of its position or state, e.g., as in a compressed spring.

**34. A rocket releases a satellite into orbit around Earth. The satellite travels at 2000 m/s in 25 seconds. What is the acceleration?**

a. 60 m/sec$^2$

b. 80 m/sec$^2$

c. 100 m/sec$^2$

d. 120 m/sec$^2$

**35. Name the four states in which matter exists.**

a. Concrete, liquid, gas, and plasma

b. Solid, fluid, gas, and plasma

c. Solid, , vapor, and plasma

d. Solid, liquid, gas, and plasma

**36. Which one of the following best describes the function of a cell membrane?**

    a. It controls the substances entering and leaving the cell.

    b. It keeps the cell in shape.

    c. It controls the substances entering the cell.

    d. It supports the cell structures

**37. Describe electric current.**

    a. Electric current is the flow of voltage

    b. Electric current is the movement of negative ions.

    c. Electric current is the flow of electric charge through a medium.

    d. None of the above

**38. Which of the following is not a typical shape for a bacterium?**

    a. Rod

    b. Spiral

    c. Sphere

    d. Cube

**39. What is usually the result when acid reacts with most of the metals?**

    a. Carbon dioxide

    b. Oxygen gas

    c. Nitrogen gas

    d. Hydrogen gas

**40. Which of these is not a rank within the area of classification or taxonomy?**

    a. Species

    b. Family

    c. Genus

    d. Relative position

**41. Which of the following statements about the periodic table of the elements is true?**

a. On the periodic table, the elements are arranged according to their atomic mass.

b. The way in which the elements are arranged allows for predictions to made about their behavior.

c. The vertical columns of the table are called rows.

d. The horizontal rows of the table are called groups.

**42. The scientific term _____ refers to a practical test designed with the intention that its results be relevant to a particular theory or set of theories.**

a. Procedure

b. Variable

c. Hypothesis

d. Experiment

**43. Substances that deactivate catalysts are called**

a. Inhibitors

b. Catalytic poisons

c. Positive catalysts

d. None of the above

**44. What is the force per unit area exerted against a surface by the weight of air above that surface in the Earth's atmosphere?**

a. Gravitational force

b. Atmospheric pressure

c. Barometric density

d. Aneroid pressure

## 45. Describe kinetic energy.

a. Kinetic energy is the energy an object possesses due to its mass.

b. Kinetic energy is the energy an object possesses due to its motion.

c. Kinetic energy is the energy an object possesses due to its chemical properties.

d. Kinetic energy is the stored energy an object possesses.

## 46. Another term for biological classification is:

a.  Darwinian classification

b.  Animal classification

c.  Molecular classification

d.  Scientific classification

## 47. When do oxidation and reduction reactions occur?

a. One after the other

b. In separate reactions

c. On the product side of the reaction

d. Simultaneously

## 48. What type of gene is not expressed as a trait unless inherited by both parents?

a. Principal gene

b. Latent gene

c. Recessive gene

d. Dominant gene

**49. A _____ _____ is an approximation or simulation of a real system that omits all but the most essential variables of the system.**

    a. Scientific method

    b. Independent variable

    c. Control group

    d. Scientific model

**50. A proton is:**

    a. A subatomic particle that forms part of the nucleus on an atom.

    b. The nucleus of an atom.

    c. An atomic particle that forms part of the nucleus on an atom.

    d. A microscopic particle that forms part of the nucleus on an atom.

**51. Neutrons are necessary within an atomic nucleus because**

    a. They bind with protons via nuclear force

    b. They bind with nuclei via nuclear force

    c. They bind with protons via electromagnetic force

    d. They bind with nuclei via electromagnetic force

**52. How do atoms of different elements combine to form chemical mixtures?**

    a. Atoms of different elements combine in simple whole-number ratios to form chemical compounds.

    b. Atoms of different components combine in simple fractional ratios to form chemical compounds.

    c. Atoms of the same element combine in simple whole-number ratios to form chemical compounds.

    d. Atoms of different elements combine in simple whole-number ratios to form chemical mixtures.

## 53. Which of the following statements is false?

a. Most enzymes are proteins

b. Enzymes are catalysts

c. Most enzymes are inorganic

d. Enzymes are large biological molecules

## 54. _____ are compounds that contain hydrogen, can dissolve in water to release hydrogen ions into solution, and, in an aqueous solution, can conduct electricity.

a. Caustics

b. Bases

c. Acids

d. Salts

## 55. Find the momentum of a round stone weighing 12.05 kg rolling down a hill at 8 m/s.

a.  95 kg m/sec down the hill.

b.  96.4 kg m/sec down the hill.

c.  100 kg m/sec down the hill.

d.  90 kg m/sec down the hill.

## 56. Which of the following statements about non-metals are false?

a. A non-metal is a substance that conducts heat and electricity poorly.

b. Most known chemical elements are non-metals.

c. A non-metal is brittle or waxy or gaseous.

d. None of the statements are false.

**57. What is the name of the discipline that studies bacteria?**

    a. Bacteriography

    b. Bacteriology

    c. Bacteriepathy

    d. Bacterioscopy

**58. What are the basic structural units of nucleic acids (DNA or RNA) whose sequence determines individual hereditary characteristics?**

    a. Gene

    b. Nucleotide

    c. Phosphate

    d. Nitrogen base

**59. Which of these statements about light energy is/ are true?**

    a. Light consists of electromagnetic waves in the visible range.

    b. The fundamental particle or quantum of light is a photon.

    c. A and B are true.

    d. None of the statements are true.

**60. List the classifications of organisms in order of size.**

    a. Genus, Kingdom, Phylum/division, Class, Order, and Family Species

    b. Order, Kingdom, Phylum/division, Genus, Class, and Family Species

    c. Genus, Kingdom, Phylum/division, Class, Order, and Family Species

    d. Kingdom ,Genus, Phylum/division, Class, Order, and Family Species

    e. Family species, Order, Class, Phylum/division, Kingdom, and Genus

## 61. Explain chemical bonds.

a. Chemical bonds are attractions between atoms that form chemical substances containing two or more atoms.

b. Chemical bonds are attractions between protons that form chemical elements containing two or more atoms.

c. Chemical bonds are two or more atoms that form chemical substances.

d. None of the above

## 62. The number of protons in the nucleus of an atom is the

a. Atomic mass.

b. Atomic weight.

c. Atomic number.

d. None of the above.

## 63. The molarity of an aqueous solution of CaCl is defined as the

a. moles of CaCl per milliliter of solution

b. grams of CaCl per liter of water

c. grams of CaCl per milliliter of solution

d. moles of CaCl per liter of solution

## 64. An electron is:

a. A tiny particle with a negative charge.

b. A tiny particle with a positive charge.

c. A tiny particle with a negative charge that orbits a nucleus.

d. A tiny particle with a positive charge that orbits an atom.

**65. What law states that, in a chemical change, energy can be neither created nor destroyed, but only changed from one form to another?**

    a. The Law of the Preservation of Matter

    b. The Law of the Conservation of Energy

    c. The Law of the Conservation of Energy

    d. The Law of the Conservation of Energy

**66. What is the simplest unit of any compound?**

    a. Atom

    b. Proton

    c. Molecule

    d. Compound

**67. Sex chromosomes are designated as being "X" or "Y" chromosomes. In terms of sex chromosomes, what differences exist between males and females?**

    a. Females have two X chromosomes and males have one X chromosome and one Y chromosome.

    b. Females have one X chromosome, and males have one X chromosome and one Y chromosome.

    c. Females have one Y chromosome, while males have one X chromosome.

    d. Females have one X chromosome and one Y chromosome, and males have two X chromosomes.

**68. A biofilm is**

    a. A dense aggregation of bacteria attached to surfaces.

    b. A type of bacteria which causes disease.

    c. A cluster of bacteria which is healthy to consume.

    d. Bacteria which aids in digestion.

## 69. Identify the chemical properties of water.

a. Water has two hydrogen atoms covalently bonded to one oxygen atom.

b. Water has two oxygen atoms covalently bonded to one hydrogen atom.

c. Water has two hydrogen atoms polar covalently bonded to one oxygen atom.

d. Water has two oxygen atoms polar covalently bonded to one hydrogen atom.

## 70. What unit is electrical resistance measured?

a. Ohms

b. Volts

c. Amps

d. None of the above

## 71. Calculate the molarity of 2.5 liters of a lithium fluoride, LiF solution that contains 52 grams of LiF.
## (Gram-formula - atomic mass = 26 grams/mole)

a. 0.8 M

b. 1.5 M

c. 0.5 mol

d. 2 mol

## 72. In physics, _____ is the force that opposes the relative motion of two bodies in contact.

a. Resistance

b. Abrasiveness

c. Friction

d. Antagonism

**73. What is the difference between anabolism and catabolism?**

    a. Anabolism is the series of chemical reactions resulting in the synthesis of inorganic compounds, and catabolism is a series of chemical reactions that break down larger molecules.

    b. Anabolism is the series of chemical reactions resulting in the synthesis of organic compounds, and catabolism is a series of chemical reactions that combine larger molecules.

    c. Catabolism is the series of chemical reactions resulting in the synthesis of organic compounds, and anabolism is a series of chemical reactions that break down larger molecules.

    d. Anabolism is the series of chemical reactions resulting in the synthesis of organic compounds, and catabolism is a series of chemical reactions that break down larger molecules.

**74. What results when acid reacts with a base?**

    a. A weak acid

    b. A weak base

    c. A salt and water

    d. Hydrogen

**75. What is a reaction where an element gains electrons known as?**

    a. Reduction

    b. Oxidation

    c. Sublimation

    d. Condensation

# Section VI - Anatomy and Physiology

**1. The quadrant that is largely responsible for digestion is _____.**

    a. Left Upper

    b. Right Upper

    c. Right Lower

    d. Left Lower

**2. Human homeostasis is the ability of the body to regulate its _____ in response to fluctuations in the environment outside the body.**

    a. Inner environment

    b. Outer environment

    c. Temperature

    d. Metabolism

**3. An important function of epithelial tissue is**

    a. Strengthen the muscles.

    b. Acting as a protective barrier for the human body.

    c. Protect the nerves.

    d. Nonexistent; it has been found to have no known function.

**4. The bodily organ system which protects the person's body from damage is the _____ system.**

    a. Circulatory

    b. Musculoskeletal

    c. Integumentary

    d. Digestive

## 5. Another primary purpose of the musculoskeletal system is

a. Moving oxygen

b. Cleansing the blood stream

c. Relaxing the mind

d. Providing form for the body

## 6. What are examples of nutrients passed along via the circulatory system?

a. Citric acids

b. Amino acids

c. Proteins

d. Nuclei

## 7. Which of the following is an example of an important component of the respiratory system?

a. The cornea

b. The lungs

c. The kidneys

d. The stomach

## 8. How does the immune system fight off disease?

a. By identifying and killing tumor cells and pathogens.

b. By creating new blood cells that fight disease.

c. By expelling infection through the blood stream.

d. By giving you energy to resist disease infections.

## 9. What is the primary purpose of the digestive system?

a. To expel food and liquids from the body.

b. To absorb oxygen from food.

c. To help circulate blood throughout the body.

d. To convert food into a form that can provide nourishment for the body.

## 10. What is mostly true of urine?

a. It's mostly comprised of healthy vitamins and nutrients.

b. It's mostly comprised of waste material after the body has taken the nutrients from food and absorbed the water it needs.

c. It's mostly useless in the body.

d. It's mostly carbohydrates.

## 11. The gallbladder is located in the

a. RUQ

b. LUQ

c. LLQ

d. RLQ

## 12. The lymphatic system is defined as the system which

a. Carries a clear liquid ("lymph") toward the heart.

b. Carries a clear liquid ("lymph") out through the bowels.

c. Heals the lymph nodes.

d. Cleanses the blood stream of bacteria.

## 13. Which organ of the body acts as a biological filter of blood?

a. The spleen

b. Bone marrow

c. The liver

d. The heart

**14. The body organ that is NOT located within the Right Upper Quadrant is**

a. Liver

b. Gall Bladder

c. Duodenum

d. Sigmoid colon

**15. An example of a person whose metabolism has lowered is**

a. A woman who is in her teens and quite athletic.

b. A man who is past 30 and whose body is losing muscle.

c. A man who is past 30 and works out daily.

d. A man who is past 30 and eats a low-fat diet.

**16. Muscle tissue can _____, bringing out movement and the ability to work.**

a. Divide and conquer

b. Replicate at will

c. Relax and contract

d. Sleep

**17. How many layers of skin are contained within the human integumentary system (skin)?**

a. One

b. Two

c. Three

d. Four

## 18. What is cartilage?

a. A flexible, connective tissue that keeps bones from rubbing against each other

b. The material that comprises the brain

c. A part of human blood responsible for fighting infection

d. Another name for the femur

## 19. What are the main components of the circulatory system?

a. The heart, veins and blood vessels

b. The heart, brain, and ears

c. The nose, throat and ears

d. The lungs, stomach, and kidneys

## 20. The exchange of oxygen for carbon dioxide takes place in the alveolar area of

a. The throat

b. The ears

c. The appendix

d. The lungs

## 21. Detection of pathogens can be complicated because

a. They evolve so quickly

b. They die so quickly

c. They are invisible

d. They multiply so quickly

**22. Which of these is not an example of a function of the stomach in digestion?**

    a. Storing food

    b. Cleansing food of impurities

    c. Mixing food with digestive juices

    d. Transferring food into the intestines

**23. What is the name of the waste removed from the body through urine?**

    a. Urea

    b. Urinalysis

    c. Feces

    d. Fat

**24. An example of an organ that plays a big role in the lymphatic system is**

    a. The spine

    b. The kidney

    c. The spleen

    d. The liver

**25. What controls reflex action?**

    a. The sympathetic nervous system

    b. The parasympathetic nervous system.

    c. The central nervous system

    d. The sensory nerves

# Answer Key

# Section 1 – Reading Comprehension

### 1. A
Helen's parents hired Anne to teach Helen to communicate. Choice B is incorrect because the passage states Anne had trouble finding her way around, which means she could walk. **Choic**e C is incorrect because you don't hire a teacher to teach someone to play. Choice D is incorrect because by age 6, if Helen had never eaten, she would have starved to death.

### 2. B
The correct answer because that fact is stated directly in the passage. The passage explains that Anne taught Helen to hear by allowing her to feel the vibrations in her throat.

### 3. A
We can **inf**er that Anne is a patient teacher because she did not leave or lose her temper when Helen bit or hit her; she just kept trying to teach Helen. Choice B is incorrect because Anne taught Helen to read and talk. Choice C is incorrect because Anne could hear. She was partially blind, not deaf. Choice D is incorrect because it does not have to do with patience.

### 4. B
The pa**ssag**e states that it was hard for anyone but Anne to understand Helen when she spoke. Choice A is incorrect because the passage does not mention Helen spoke a foreign language. Choice C is incorrect because there is no mention of how quiet or loud Helen's voice was. Choice D is incorrect because we know from reading the passage that Helen did learn to speak.

### 5. D
This question tests the reader's summarization skills. The question is asking very generally about the message of the passage, and the title, "Ways Characters Communicate in Theater," is one indication of that. The other choices A, B,

and C are all directly from the text, and therefore readers may be inclined to select one of them, but are too specific to encapsulate the entirety of the passage and its message.

## 6. B

The paragraph on soliloquies mentions "To be or not to be," and it is from the context of that paragraph that readers may understand that because "To be or not to be" is a soliloquy, Hamlet will be introspective, or thoughtful, while delivering it. It is true that actors deliver soliloquies alone, and may be "solitary" (choice A), but "thoughtful" (choice B) is more true to the overall idea of the paragraph. Readers may choose C because drama and theater can be used interchangeably and the passage mentions that soliloquies are unique to theater (and therefore drama), but this answer is not specific enough to the paragraph in question. Readers may pick up on the theme of life and death and Hamlet's true intentions and select that he is "hopeless" (choice D), but those themes are not discussed either by this paragraph or passage, as a close textual reading and analysis confirms.

## 7. C

This question tests the reader's grammatical skills. Choice B seems logical, but parenthesis are actually considered to be a stronger break in a sentence than commas are, and along this line of thinking, actually disrupt the sentence more.

Choices A and D make comparisons between theater and film that are simply not made in the passage, and may or may not be true. This detail does clarify the statement that asides are most unique to theater by adding that it is not completely unique to theater, which may have been why the author didn't chose not to delete it and instead used parentheses to designate the detail's importance (choice C).

**8. A**
Low blood sugar occurs both in diabetics and healthy adults.

**9. B**
None of the statements are the author's opinion.

**10. A**
The author's purpose is the inform.

**11. A**
The only statement that is not a detail is, "A doctor can diagnosis this medical condition by asking the patient questions and testing."

**12. A**
This sentence is a recommendation.

**13. C**
Tips for a good night's sleep is the best alternative title for this article.

**14. B**
Mental activity is helpful for a good night's sleep is can not be inferred from this article.

**15. A**
From the passage, one disadvantage of taking naps is they may keep you awake at night.

**16. C**
Based on the partial table of contents, you would find information about natural selection in the ecology section on page 110.

**17. C**
To be infamous means to be remembered for an evil or terrible action. Therefore, the word infamy means to remember a bad or terrible thing. Choice A is incorrect because being famous is not the same as being infamous. Choice B is incorrect because the attack on Pearl Harbor was not good. Choice D is incorrect because Pearl Harbor was not forgotten.

**18. C**
Each other answer set contains the name of at least one country that was not part of the AXIS powers.

**19. D**
It is stated in the passage. Choice A is not correct because there was no indication that Japan would attack San Diego Choice B is incorrect because the attack on Pearl Harbor was a surprise. Choice C is incorrect because Roosevelt was not planning to attack Japan.

**20. C**
The passage clearly states that Japan planned a surprise attack. They chose that early time to catch the U.S. military off guard. Choice A is incorrect because the military does not sleep late. Choice B is incorrect because there is no law against bombing countries. Choice D is incorrect because it makes no sense.

**21. C**
This question tests the reader's vocabulary skills. The uses of the negatives "but" and "less," especially right next to each other, may confuse readers into answering with choices A or D, which list words that are antonyms to "militant." Readers may also be confused by the comparison of healthy people with what is being described as an overly healthy person--both people are good, but the reader may look for which one is "worse" in the comparison, and therefore stray toward the antonym words. One key to understanding the meaning of "militant" if the reader is unfamiliar with it is to look at the root of the word; readers can then easily associate it with "military" and gain a sense of what the word signifies: defence (especially considered that the immune system defends the body). Choice C is correct over choice B because "militant" is an adjective, just as the words in choice C are, whereas the words in choice B are nouns.

**22. C**
This question tests the reader's understanding of function within writing. The other choices are details included surrounding the quoted text, and may therefore confuse the reader. Choice A somewhat contradicts what is said

earlier in the paragraph, which is that tests and treatments are improving, and probably doctors are along with them, but the paragraph doesn't actually mention doctors, and the subject of the question is the medicine. Choice B may seem correct to readers who aren't careful to understand that, while the author does mention the large number of people affected, the author is touching on the realities of living with allergies, rather than the likelihood of curing all allergies. Similarly, while the author does mention the "balance" of the body, which is easily associated with "wholesome," the author is not really making an argument and especially is not making an extreme statement that allergy medicines should be outlawed. Again, because the article's tone is on living with allergies, choice C is an appropriate choice that fits with the title and content of the text.

**23. B**
This question tests the reader's inference skills. The text does not state who is doing the recommending, but the use of the "patients," as well as the general context of the passage, lends itself to the logical partner, "doctors," choice B. The author does mention the recommendation but doesn't present it as her own (i.e. "I recommend that"), so choice A may be eliminated. It may seem plausible that people with allergies (choice D) may recommend medicines or products to other people with allergies, but the text does not necessarily support this interaction taking place. Choice C may be selected because the EpiPen is specifically mentioned, but the use of the phrase "such as" when it is introduced is not limiting enough to assume the recommendation is coming from its creators.

**24. D**
This question tests the reader's global understanding of the text. Choice D includes the main topics of the three body paragraphs, and isn't too focused on a specific aspect or quote from the text, as the other questions are, giving a skewed summary of what the author intended. The reader may be drawn to choice B because of the title of the passage and the use of words like "better," but the message of the passage is larger and more general than this.

## 25. B
Reading the document posted to the Human Resources website is optional.

## 26. B
The document is recommended changes and have not be implemented yet.

## 27. C
This question tests the reader's summarization skills. The use of the word "actually" in describing what kind of people poets are, as well as other moments like this, may lead readers to selecting choices B or D, but the author is more information than trying to persuade readers. The author gives no indication that she loves poetry (choice B) or that people, students specifically (D), should write poems. Choice A is incorrect because the style and content of this paragraph do not match those of a foreword; forewords usually focus on the history or ideas of a specific poem to introduce it more fully and help it stand out against other poems. The author here focuses on several poems and gives broad statements. Instead, she tells a kind of story about poems, giving three very broad time periods in which to discuss them, thereby giving a brief history of poetry, as choice C states.

## 28. A
This question tests the reader's summarization skills. Key words in the topic sentences of each of the paragraphs ("oldest," "Renaissance," "modern") should give the reader an idea that the author is moving chronologically. The opening and closing sentence-paragraphs are broad and talk generally. B seems reasonable, but epic poems are mentioned in two paragraphs, eliminating the idea that only new types of poems are used in each paragraph. Choice C is also easily eliminated because the author clearly mentions several different poets, groups of people, and poems. Choice D also seems reasonable, considering that the author does move from older forms of poetry to newer forms, but use of "so (that)" makes this statement false, for the author gives no indication that she is rushing (the paragraphs are about the same size) or that she prefers modern poetry.

## 29. D
This question tests the reader's attention to detail. The key word is "invented"-- it ties together the Mesopotamians, who invented the written word, and the fact that they, as the inventors, also invented and used poetry. The other selections focus on other details mentioned in the passage, such as that the Renaissance's admiration of the Greeks (choice C) and that Beowulf is in Old English (choice A). Choice B may seem like an attractive answer because it is unlike the others and because the idea of heroes seems rooted in ancient and early civilizations.

## 30. B
This question tests the reader's vocabulary and contextualization skills. "Telling" is not an unusual word, but it may be used here in a way that is not familiar to readers, as an adjective rather than a verb in gerund form. A may seem like the obvious answer to a reader looking for a verb to match the use they are familiar with. If the reader understands that the word is being used as an adjective and that choice A is a ploy, they may opt to select choice D, "wordy," but it does not make sense in context. Choice C can be easily eliminated, and doesn't have any connection to the paragraph or passage. "Significant" (choice B) makes sense contextually, especially relative to the phrase "give insight" used later in the sentence.

## 31. C
Wind is the highest source of renewable energy in Scotland. The other choices are either not mentioned at all or not mentioned in the context for how fast they are growing.

## 32. A
Most Scottish citizens agree with the Government's plan due to the concern for current and future needs.

Choice B is a good choice but not why the majority agree. Choice C is meant to mislead the as they are clearly in sight. Choice D is a good 'common sense' choice but mentioned specifically in the text.

## 33. C
The up-front cost is expensive.

The other choices may appear to be correct, and even be common sense, but they are not specifically mentioned in the paragraph.

**34. D**
The best way to describe the paragraphs description of wind energy is clean and renewable but fluctuating.
The other choices are good descriptions of wind energy, but not the best way to describe the article.

**35. A**
The Save the Children's fund has raised $12,000 out of $20,000, or 12/20. Simplifying, 12/20 = 3/5

# Section II – Mathematics
**1. A**
1/3 X 3/4 = 3/12 = 1/4

**2. D**
75/1500 = 15/300 = 3/60 = 1/20

**3. D**
3.14 + 2.73 = 5.87 and 5.87 + 23.7 = 29.57

**4. B**
Spent 15% - 100% - 15% = 85%

**5. C**
To convert a decimal to a fraction, take the places of decimal as your denominator, in this case 2, so in 0.27, '7' is in the 100th place, so the fraction is 27/100 and 0.33 becomes 33/100.

Next estimate the answer quickly to eliminate obvious wrong choices. 27/100 is about 1/4 and 33/100 is 1/3. 1/3 is slightly larger than 1/4, and 1/4 + 1/4 is 1/2, so the answer will be slightly larger than 1/2.

Looking at the choices, Choice A can be eliminated since 3/6 = 1/2. Choice D, 2/7 is less than 1/2 and can be eliminated. So the answer is going to be Choice B or Choice C.

Do the calculation, 0.27 + 0.33 = 0.60 and 0.60 = 60/100 = 3/5, Choice C is correct.

**6. D**
3.13 + 7.87 = 11 and 11 X 5 = 55

**7. B**
2/4 X 3/4 = 6/16, and lowest terms = 3/8

**8. D**
2/3 - 2/5 = 10 - 6/15 = 4/15

**9. C**
2/7 + 2/3 = 6+14 /21 (21 is the common denominator) = 20/21

**10. B**
2/3 x 60 = 40 and 1.5 x 75 = 15, 40 + 15 = 55

**11. C**
This is an easy question, and shows how you can solve some questions without doing the calculations. The question is, 8 is what percent of 40. Take easy percentages for an approximate answer and see what you get.

10% is easy to calculate because you can drop the zero, or move the decimal point. 10% of 40 = 4, and 8 = 2 X 4, so, 8 must be 2 X 10% = 20%.

Here are the calculations which confirm the quick approximation.
8/40 = X/100 = 8 * 100 / 40X = 800/40 = X = 20

**12. D**
This is the same type of question which illustrates another method to solve quickly without doing the calculations. The question is, 9 is what percent of 36?

Ask, what is the relationship between 9 and 36? 9 X 4 = 36 so they are related by a factor of 4. If 9 is related to 36 by a factor of 4, then what is related to 100 (to get a percent) by a factor of 4?

To visualize:

9 X 4 = 36
Z X 4 = 100

So the answer is 25.  9 has the same relation to 36 as 25 has to 100.

Here are the calculations which confirm the quick approximation.
9/36 = X/100 = 9 * 100 / 36X = 900/36 = 25%.

**13. C**
3/10 * 90 = 3 * 90/10 = 27

**14. B**
.4/100 * 36 = .4 * 36/100 = .144

**15. A**
5 mg/10/mg X 1 tab/1 = .5 tablets

**16. B**
Step 1: Set up the formula to calculate the dose to be given in mg as per weight of the child:-
Dose ordered X Weight in Kg  = Dose to be given
Step 2: 20 mg  X 12 kg = 240 mg
240 mg/80 mg X 1 tab/1 = 240/80 = 3 tablets

**17. A**
Set up the formula to calculate the dose to be given in mg as per weight of the child:-
Dose ordered X Weight in Kg  = Dose to be given
Step 2: 20 mg  X 20 kg = 400 mg  (Convert 44 lb to Kg, 1 lb = 0.4536 kg, hence 44 lb = 19.95 kg approx. 20 kg)
400 mg/80 mg X 1 tab/1 = 400/80 = 5 tablets

**18. B**
3000 units/5000 units X 1 ml/1 = 3000/5000 = 0.6 ml

**19. C**
60 mg/80 mg X 1 ml/1 = 60/80 = 0.75 ml

**20. A**
Dose ordered X Weight in Kg  = Dose to be given
16 mg  X 15 kg = 240 mg
240 mg/80 mg X 1 tab/1 = 240/80 = 3 tablets

**21. C**
(Convert 1 g = 1000 mg)
1000 mg/1000 mg X 1 tsp/1 = 1000/1000 = 1 tsp

**22. D**
10 units/200 units X 1 ml/1 = 10/200 = 0.05 ml

**23. B**
$(4)(3)^3 = (4)(27) = 108$

**24. A**
1000g = 1kg., 0.007 = 1000 x 0.007 = 7g.

**25. C**
4 quarts = 1 gallon, 16 quarts = 16/4 = 4 gallons

**26. C**
1 teaspoon = 4.93 milliliters (U.S.), 2 tp = 4.93 x 2 = 9.86 ml.

**27. D**
1,000 meters = 1 kilometer, 200 m = 200/1,000 = 0.2 km.

**28. B**
12 inches = 1 ft., 72 inches = 72/12 = 6 feet

**29. C**
1 yard = 3 feet, 3 yards = 3 feet x 3 = 9 feet

**30. B**
0.45 kg = 1 pound, 1 kg. = 1/0.45 and 45 kg = 1/0.45 x 45 = 45 = 100 pounds.

**31. C**
1 g = 1,000 mg. 0.63 g = 0.63 x 1,000 = 630 mg.

## 32. D
To solve for x,
5x – 7x + 3 = -1
5x – 7x = -1 -3
-2x = -4
x = -4/ -2
x = 2

## 33. C
To solve for x, first simplify the equation
5x + 2x + 14 = 14x – 7
7x + 14 = 4x -7
7x – 14x + 14 = -7
7x – 14x = -7 – 14
-7x = -21
x = -21/-7
x=3

## 34. A
5z + 5 = 3z +6 + 11
5z -3z + 5 =6 + 11
5z – 3z = 6 + 11 -5
2z = 17 – 5
2z = 12
z= 12/2
z= 6

## 35. C
5z + 5 = 3z +6 + 11
5z -3z + 5 =6 + 11
5z – 3z = 6 + 11 -5
2z = 17 – 5
2z = 12
z= 12/2
z= 6

## 36. D
Price increased by $5 ($25-$20). The percent increase is
5/20 x 100 = 500/20 = 25%.

## 37. C
Price decreased by $5 ($25-$20). The percent decrease =
5/25 x 100 = 5 x 4 =20%.

**38. D**

30/100 x 150 = 3 x 15 = 45 (increase in number of correct answers). So the number of correct answers in second test = 150 + 45 = 195

**39. B**

Let total number of players = X

Let the number of players with long hair=Y and the number of players with short hair=Z

Then X = 4 + Z

Y = 12% of X

Z = X - 4

12.5% of X = 4

Converting from decimal to fraction gives 12.5% = 125/10 x 1/100 = 125/1000, therefore 12.5% of = 125/1000X = 4

Solve for X by multiplying both sides by 1000/125, X = 4 x 1000/125 = 32

Z = x − 4

Z = 32 − 4

z or number of short haired players = 28

**40. D**

2 glasses are broken for 43 customers so 1 glass breaks for every 43/2 customers served, therefore 10 glasses implies (43/2) * 10 = 215 customers.

**41. D**

As the lawn is square, the length of one side will be the square root of the area. √62,500 = 250 meters. So, the perimeter is found by 4 times the length of the side of the square:

250 * 4 = 1000 meters.

Since each meter costs $5.5, the total cost of the fence will be 1000 * 5.5 = $5,500.

**42. D**

The price of all the single items is same and there are 13 total items. So the total cost will be 13 × 1.3 = $16.9. After 3.5 percent tax this amount will become 16.9 × 1.035 = $17.5.

**43. C**
Area of the square = 12 × 12 = 144 cm²
Let x be the width, then 2x be the length of rectangle, so its
area will be $2x^2$ and perimeter will be 2(2x + x) = 6x
According to the condition
$2x^2$ = 144
X = 8.48 cm
The perimeter will be
Perimeter = 6 × 8.48
= 50.88
= 51 cm.

**44. B**
There are 50 balls in the basket now. Let x be the number
of yellow balls to be added to make 65%. So the equation
becomes

X + 15 /X + 50 = 65/100
X = 50

**45. D**
Let x be number of rows, and number of trees in a row. So
equation becomes
$X^2$ = 65536
X = 256

**46. A**
The distribution is done in three different rates and
amounts:

$6.4 per 20 kilograms to 15 shops ... 20 * 15 = 300
kilograms distributed

$3.4 per 10 kilograms to 12 shops ... 10 * 12 = 120
kilograms distributed

550 - (300 + 120) = 550 - 420 = 130 kilograms left. This
amount is distributed by 5 kilogram portions. So, this
means that there are 130/5 = 26 shops.

$1.8 per 130 kilograms.

We need to find the amount he earned overall these
distributions.

$6.4 per 20 kilograms : 6.4 * 15 = $96 for 300 kilograms

$3.4 per 10 kilograms : 3.4 * 12 = $40.8 for 120 kilograms

$1.8 per 5 kilograms : 1.8 * 26 = $46.8 for 130 kilograms

So, he earned 96 + 40.8 + 46.8 = $ 183.6

The total cost of distribution is given as $10

The profit is found by: Money earned - money spent ... It is important to remember that he bought 550 kilograms of potatoes for $165 at the beginning:

Profit = 183.6 - 10 - 165 = $8.6

**47. D**
Each tree will require a 10-meter diametric space around its stem. So 65 trees can be planted along 650-meter side. Similarly, 65 along the other side. However, along the 780 meter side, the first tree will be after 10 meters at both edges, so 76 trees can be planted long that side.

Total number of trees then will be 65×2+76×2=282

**48. D**
1 foot is equal to 12 inches. So 1 ft$^2$ = 12 * 12 in$^2$

4 ft$^2$ = 4 * 12 * 12 in$^2$ = 576 in$^2$

The surface area is divided equally among 3 boys.

Each boy will clean 576/3 = 192 in$^2$

192 in$^2$ = 144 in$^2$ + 48 in$^2$; 144 in$^2$ = 1 ft$^2$

So, each boy will clean 1 ft$^2$ and 48 in$^2$

**49. B**
We check the fractions taking place in the question. We see that there is a "half" (that is 1/2) and 3/7. So, we multiply the denominators of these fractions to decide how to name the total money. We say that Mr. Johnson has 14x at the beginning; he gives half of this, meaning 7x, to his family.

$250 to his landlord. He has 3/7 of his money left. 3/7 of 14x is equal to:

14x * (3/7) = 6x

So,

Spent money is: 7x + 250

Unspent money is: 6x

Total money is: 14x

We write an equation: total money = spent money + unspent money

14x = 7x + 250 + 6x

14x - 7x - 6x = 250

x = 250

We are asked to find the total money that is 14x:

14x = 14 * 250 = $3500

**50. A**
The probability that the 1st ball drawn is red = 4/11
The probability that the 2nd ball drawn is green = 5/10
The combined probability will then be 4/11 X 5/10 = 20/110 = 2/11

# Section III English Grammar

**1. A**
The third conditional is used for talking about an unreal situation (a situation that did not happen) in the past. For example, "If I had studied harder, [if clause] I would have passed the exam" [main clause]. This has the same meaning as, "I failed the exam, because I didn't study hard enough."

**2. A**
A Pronoun should conform to its antecedent in gender, number and person.

**3. C**
The verb might is used to express possibility or permission when in the past tense. May is the present tense of might.

**4. C**
In double negative sentences, one negative is replaced with "any."

**5. C**
Words such as neither, each, many, either, every, everyone, everybody and any should take a singular pronoun.

**6. C**
The present perfect tense cannot be used with specific time expressions such as yesterday, one year ago, last week, when I was a child, at that moment, that day, one day, etc. The present perfect tense is used with unspecific expressions such as ever, never, once, many times, several times, before, so far, already, yet, etc.

**7. A**
"Went" is used in the simple past tense. "Gone" is used in the past perfect tense.

**8. C**
Although 'can' can be used to mean the same thing as 'may,' the difference is that 'can' is used for negative or interrogative sentences, while 'may' is used in affirmative sentences to express possibility.

**9. C**
Words such as neither, each, many, either, every, everyone, everybody and any should take a singular pronoun. Here we are assuming that the subject is female, and so use "her." The subject could be male, in which case we would use "his," however that is not a choice here.

**10. C**
"It's" is a contraction for it is or it has. "Its" is a possessive pronoun.

**11. B**
The sentence refers to a person, so "who" is the only correct choice.

## 12. A
The sentence requires the past perfect "has always been known." Furthermore, this is the only grammatically correct choice.

## 13. B
"Will" is used in the second or third person (they, he, she and you), while "shall" is used in the first person (I and we). Both verbs are used to express futurity. In common usage and everyday conversation, however, they can be interchanged.

## 14. D
When comparing two items, use "the taller." When comparing more than two items, use "the tallest."

## 15. B
The past perfect form is used to describe an event that occurred in the past and prior to another event. Here there are two things that happened, both of them in the past, and something the person wanted to do.

Event 1: Kiss came to town
Event 2: All the tickets sold out
What I wanted to do: Buy a ticket

The events are arranged:

When KISS came to town, all the tickets had been sold out before I could buy one.

## 16. A
The subject is "rules" so the present tense plural form, "are," is used to agree with "realize."

## 17. A
Use "whom" in the objective case, and use "who" a subjective case.

## 18. D
The simple past tense, "sank," is correct because it refers to completed action in the past.

**19. A**
"Who" is correct because the question uses an active construction. "To whom was first place given?" is passive construction.

**20. D**
"Which" is correct, because the files are objects and not people.

**21. C**
The simple present tense, "rises," is correct.

**22. A**
"Lie" does not require a direct object, while "lay" does. The old woman might lie on the couch, which has no direct object, or she might lay the book down, which has the direct object, "the book."

**23. D**
The simple present tense, "falls," is correct because it is repeated action.

**24. A**
The present progressive, "building models," is correct in this sentence; it is required to match the other present progressive verbs.

**25. A**
"Affect" is a verb, while "effect" is a noun.

**26. D**
"Than" is used for comparison. "Then" is used to show a point in time.

**27. C**
"There" shows a state of existence. "Their" is used for third person plural possession. "They're" is the contracted form of "they are."

**28. A**
The verb "ought" expresses desirability, duty and probability. The verb is usually followed by "to."

**29. A**

When you use 'each other' it should be used for two things or people. When you use 'one another' it should be used for more than two things or people.

**30. C**

"Your" is the possessive form of "you." "You're" is the contraction of "you are."

**31. A**

Disease is a singular noun.

**32. C**

Both "dog" and "cat" in this sentence are singular nouns and require the article "a."

**33. A**

The word "principal" is a synonym for primary or major. "Principle" means a fundamental truth.

**34. D**

The article "a" come before a noun that begins with a consonant, while "an" comes before a noun that begins with a vowel.

**35. A**

"Except" means to exclude something. "Accept" means to receive something, or to agree to an idea.

**36. A**

"Advise" is a verb that means to offer advice, which is a noun.

**37. C**

"Adapt" means to change or accommodate. "Adopt" means to accept, embrace, or to assume responsibility or ownership for something or someone.

**38. D**

"Among" is used with more than two items, while "between" is limited to two items.

**39. D**
"At" refers to a specific time or location, while "about" is approximate.

**40. B**
"Beside" means next to, and "besides" means in addition to.

**41. A**
"Can" is used when describing ability or capability. "May" is a request or the granting of permission.

**42. B**
"Continuous" means a time period without interruption, or ongoing. "Continual" is used for actions that are frequent and repetitive, or that continue almost without interruption.

**43. A**
"Emigrate" means to leave one's country, usually to immigrate to another country to live.

**44. A**
"Farther" is reserved for physical distance, and "further" is used for figurative distance, or to mean "in addition."

**45. B**
"Former" refers to the first of two things; "latter" to the second of two things.

**46. D**
"Healthy" describes people or animals that are in good health. "Healthful" is generally used in formal speech or writing, and refers to things that are good for health.

**47. C**
"Lie" does not require a direct object, while "lay" does. In this sentence, "lay" is followed by the direct object, "the books."

**48. C**
"Lie" does not require a direct object, while "lay" does. In this sentence, "lay" is followed by the direct object, "the books."

**49. C**
This is the correct choice.

**50. A**
"Learn" means to receive and integrate knowledge or an experience. "Teach" means to impart knowledge to another.

# Section IV Vocabulary

**1. C**
**Dauntless:** adj. Invulnerable to fear or intimidation.

**2. A**
**Juxtaposed:** adj. Placed side-by-side often for comparison or contrast.

**3. B**
**Regicide:** v. killing of a king.

**4. A**
**Pernicious:** adj. Causing much harm in a subtle way.

**5. A**
**Immune:** adj. Resistant to a particular infection or toxin owing to the presence of specific antibodies.

**6. B**
**Nimble:** adj. Quick and light in movement or action.

**7. A**
**Queries:** n. Questions or inquiries.

**8. C**
**Depose:** To remove (a leader) from (high) office, without killing the incumbent.

**9. D**
**Pedestrian:** Ordinary, dull; everyday; unexceptional.

**10. B**
**Petulant:** adj. Childishly irritable.

**11. D**
**Pesticide:** n. A substance used for destroying insects or other organisms harmful to cultivated plants or to animals.

**12. D**
**Salient:** adj. worthy or note or relevant.

**13. B**
**Sedentary:** adj. not moving or sitting in one place.

**14. A**
**Famine:** n. extreme scarcity of food.

**15. A**
**Stint:** n. To be sparing.

**16. A**
**Precipitate:** v. to rain.

**17. C**
**Edify:** v. To instruct or improve morally or intellectually.

**18. B**
**Egress:** n. An exit or way out.

**19. A**
**Recede:** v. To move back, to move away.

**20. A**
**Confidential:** adj. kept secret within a certain circle of persons; not intended to be known publicly.

**21. A**
**Aggravate:**  v. to make worse, or more severe; to render less tolerable or less excusable; to make more offensive; to enhance; to intensify.

**22. B**
**Debut:** n. a performer's first-time performance to the public.

**23. B**
**Hormones:**  n. A regulatory substance produced in an

organism and transported in tissue fluids such as blood or sap to stimulate specific cells.

**24. B**
**Importune:** v. To harass with persistent requests.

**25. B**
**Sedulous:** adj. Showing dedication and diligence.

**26. A**
**Tincture:** n. alcoholic drink with plant extracts used for medicine.

**27. C**
**Felony:** n. Serious criminal offence that is punishable by death or imprisonment above a year.

**28. A**
**Bibliophile**: n. One who loves books.

**29. A**
**Monsoons:** n. The rainy season accompanying the wet monsoon.

**30. D**
**Volatile:** adj. Explosive.

**31. B**
**Plaintive:** adj. Sorrowful, mournful or melancholic.

**32. B**
**Truism**: n. Self-evident or clear obvious truth.

**33. B**
**Foment:** v. to encourage or incite troublesome acts.

**34. A**
**Funereal:** Adj. dignified, solemn that is appropriate for a funeral.

**35. A**
**Flagrant:** obvious and offensive, blatant, scandalous.

**36. B**
**Moss**

**37. A**
**Nexus:** n. A connection or series of connections linking two or more things.

**38. A**
**Zealot:** n. A person who is very passionate and fanatic about his specific objectives or beliefs.

**39. B**
**Vertigo:** n. Dizziness.

**40. A**
**Trenchant:** adj. Vigorous or incisive in expression or style.

**41. B**
**Geniality:** n. warmth and kindness of disposition.

**42. A**
**Habitual:** adj. Behaving in a regular manner, as a habit.

**43. B**
**Idolize:** v. To make an idol of, or to worship as an idol.

**44. C**
**Osculate:** v. to kiss or related to kissing.

**45. D**
**Conjoin:** v. To join; to unite; to combine.

**46. B**
**Petrify:** v. To harden organic matter by permeating with water and depositing dissolved minerals.

**47. A**
**Extinguish:** v. Cause a fire or light to cease to burn or shine.

**48. C**
**Convection:** n. Heat transfer in a gas or liquid by the circulation of currents.

**49. A**
**Intrepid:** adj. Fearless; adventurous.

**50. D**
**Goad:** v. To encourage, stimulate or incite and provoke.

## Section V – Science

### 1. A
The formula for acceleration = A = $(V_f - V_0)/t$
so A = (120 -90)/5 sec = 6 mph/second²

### 2. A
Only genetics pertains directly to the cell's function. For genetics, the cell of a new organism acquires traits of an-cestral organisms.

### 3. A
A solution with a pH value of greater than 7 is base.

### 4. B
The voltage across a resistor is equal to the product of the resistance and the current flowing through it.

### 5. A
Eukaryotic and prokaryotic cells are both organelles.

### 6. C
Electric potential is a fundamental interaction between the magnetic field and the presence and motion of an electric charge.

Electric potential is the capacity of an electric field to do work on an electric charge, typically measured in volts, while electromagnetism is a fundamental interaction be-tween the magnetic field and the presence and motion of an electric charge.

### 7. C
Subversion. Active transport, adhesion and cell signaling are all involved in cellular biology.

### 8. C
Homologous is being inherited by the organisms' common ancestors. An example would be feathers and hair—both share a common ancestral trait.

**9. C**
The manner in which instructions for building proteins, the basic structural molecules of living material are written in the DNA is a **genetic code**.

**10. C**
A gene is a unit of inherited material, encoded by a strand of DNA and transcribed by RNA.

**11. B**
Speed = (total distance traveled)/(total time taken)
6 = x/120   (convert minutes to seconds)
6 * 120 = x
X = 720 meters

**12. D**
Cellular scientists' biographies are not studied in cell biology. The physiological properties of cells, cell structure and the life cycle of a cell are all valid topics of study within the field of cell biology.

**13. A**
Detection of pathogens can be complicated because they evolve so quickly.

**14. C**
Molarity = moles of solute/liters of solution = 8/4 = 2

**15. D**
An ohm (Ω) is a unit of electrical voltage is not true.

**Note:** An ohm is a unit of electrical resistance.

**16. D**
The periodic table contains 118 elements.

**17. C**
Mutations in DNA sequences usually occur spontaneously is false.

**18. C**
Momentum is a product of velocity and mass. If they are all traveling at the same speed, the car that weighs the most would have the highest momentum.

## 19. A
Starting with the weakest, the fundamental forces of nature in order of strength are, Gravity, Weak nuclear force, Electromagnetic force, Strong nuclear force.

## 20. A
Electrons are subatomic particles that carry a negative charge.

## 21. A
Cell culture is the technique for growing cells independent of a living organism within the confines of a laboratory. The cell culture is generally grown in a test-tube environment or on a petri dish.

## 22. A
Precision, which refers to the repeatability of measurement, does not require knowledge of the correct or true value.

## 23. C
All conductors contain electrical charges, which will move when an electric potential difference (measured in volts) is applied across separate points on the material. This flow of charge (measured in amperes) is what is meant by electric current.

## 24. B
The periodic table is a tabular display of the chemical elements, organized on the basis of their atomic numbers, electron configurations, and recurring chemical properties.

## 25. D
The scientific discipline that studies the physiological aspects, structures, life cycles and division of cells is called cell biology.

## 26. A
Ionization energy is the minimum amount of energy required to remove an electron from an atom or ion in the gas phase.

## 27. C
Redox is a complete reaction comprising oxidation and reduction reactions that are each only half of the complete reaction. The same exact electrons lost in oxidation are

what are gained in reduction.

**28. A**

In terms of the scientific method, the term **observation** refers to the act of noticing or perceiving something and/or recording a fact or occurrence.

**29. B**

The Lewis Theory defines acids and bases in terms of the electron-pair concept; according to its definition, an acid is an electron-pair acceptor, and a base is an electron-pair donor.

**30. A**

First convert 250 ml to liters, 250/1000 = 0.25 then calculate molarity = 5 moles/ 0.25 liters = 20 M.

**31. D**

The property of a conductor that restricts its internal flow of electrons is resistance.

**32. A**

Prokaryotic microorganisms that are usually just a few micrometers long.

**33. B**

Kinetic energy is the energy of a body that results from motion while potential energy is the energy possessed by an object by virtue of its position or state, e.g., as in a compressed spring.

**34. B**

The formula for acceleration = $A = (V_f - V_0)/t$
so A = (2000 - 0)/25 sec  = 80 m/sec$^2$

**35. D**

The four states in which matter exists are solid, liquid, gas, and plasma.

The state of matter is determined by the strength of the bonds between the atoms that make up matter.

**36. A**

The cell membrane is a selectively permeable membrane that separates the cells from the outside environment.

**37. C**
Electric current is the flow of electric charge through a medium.

**38. D**
Cubes rarely occur naturally, especially in the micro world outside of the human eye. True cubes are usually deliberately created.

**39. D**
All acids contain hydrogen. When acids react with most metals, the metals displace the hydrogen and hydrogen gas is produced.

**40. D**
Relative position. Ranks include Domain, Kingdom, Phylum, Class, Order, Family, Genus, and Species.

**41. B**
The following statements about the periodic table of the elements is true,
The way in which the elements are arranged allows for predictions to made about their behavior.

**42. D**
The scientific term **experiment** refers to a practical test designed with the intention that its results be relevant to a particular theory or set of theories.

**43. B**
Substances that deactivate catalysts are called catalytic poisons.

**44. B**
Atmospheric pressure is the force per unit area exerted against a surface by the weight of air above that surface in the Earth's atmosphere.

**45. B**
Kinetic energy is the energy an object possesses due to its motion.

**46. D**
Scientific classification. The two phrases are interchangeable, although the former seems to more accurately reflect the purpose of classification: to categorize biological units.

**47. D**
Oxidation and reduction reactions are each just half of a

redox reaction and both occur simultaneously, because the exact electrons lost in oxidation is what is gained in reduction.

**48. C**
A recessive gene is not expressed as a trait unless inherited by both parents.

**49. D**
A **scientific model** is an approximation or simulation of a real system that omits all but the most essential variables of the system.

**50. A**
A positively charged subatomic particle forming part of the nucleus of an atom and determining the atomic number of an element.

**51. A**
Neutrons are necessary within an atomic nucleus as they bind with protons via the nuclear force.

**52. A**
Atoms of different elements combine in simple whole-number ratios to form chemical compounds.

**53. C**
The following statement is false - Most enzymes are inorganic.

**54. C**
**Acids** are compounds that contain hydrogen and can dissolve in water to release hydrogen ions into solution.

**55. B**
Formula - P= kg x m/s
= 12.05kg x 8m/s
= 96.4 kg x m/s down the hill.

Note that the final answer has the proper SI unit of momentum (kg x m/s) after it and it also mentions the direction of the movement.

**56. D**
All the statements are true.

a. A non-metal is a substance that conducts heat and electricity poorly.

b. Most known chemical elements are non-metals.

c. A non-metal is brittle or waxy or gaseous.

## 57. B
The discipline that studies bacteria is Bacteriology.

## 58. A
Genes determine individual hereditary characteristics.

## 59. C
A and B are true.

a. Light consists of electromagnetic waves in the visible range.

b. The fundamental particle or quantum of light is a photon.

**Note:** Light energy is the only visible form of energy. A light bulb is a device that uses electrical energy to create electromagnetic energy in the form (in part) of visible light and heat.

## 60. A
The groups into which organisms are classified are called taxa and include, in order of size, Genus, Kingdom, Phylum/division, Class, Order, and Family Species.

## 61. A
Chemical bonds are attractions between atoms that form chemical substances containing two or more atoms.

## 62. C
In chemistry, the number of protons in the nucleus of an atom is known as the atomic number, which determines the chemical element to which the atom belongs.

## 63. D
The molarity of an aqueous solution of CaCl is defined as the moles of CaCl per liter of solution.

## 64. C
An electron is a tiny particle with a negative charge that orbits a nucleus.

## 65. C
The Law of the Conservation of Energy states that, in a chemical change, energy can be neither created nor destroyed, but only changed from one form to another.

**66. A**
An atom is the basic or fundamental unit of any matter or element.

**67. A**
Females have two X chromosomes and males have one X chromosome and one Y chromosome.

**68. A**
A biofilm is a dense aggregation of bacteria attached to surfaces. The density of these bacteria is based on many factors, such as environment, temperature, and how long they're left there undisturbed.

**69. A**
Water has two hydrogen atoms covalently bonded to one oxygen atom.

**70. A**
Electrical resistance is measured in Ohms.

**71. A**
First convert LiF grams to moles = 52 x 1/26 = 2. Now Molarity = 2 moles/2.5 liters = 0.8 M

**72. C**
In physics, friction is the force that opposes the relative motion of two bodies in contact.

**73. D**
Anabolism is the series of chemical reactions resulting in the synthesis of organic compounds, and catabolism is a series of chemical reactions that break down larger molecules.

**74. C**
When an acid and a base react, they neutralize each other's properties to form salt and water.

**75. A**
Reduction is a reaction that usually involves the gain of electrons that were lost in an oxidation reaction.

# Section VI - Anatomy and Physiology

**1. A**
The Left upper quadrant of the abdomen, is often abbreviated as LUQ, contains the stomach, spleen, left lobe of the liver, body of the pancreas, left kidney and adrenal gland.

**2. A**
Human homeostasis is the ability of the body to regulate its **inner environment** in response to fluctuations in the environment outside the body.

**3. B**
Epithelial tissue acts as a **protective barrier for the human body**.

**4. C**
The integumentary system is the organ system that protects the body from damage, comprising the skin and its appendages, including hair, scales, feathers, and nails.

**5. D**
Another primary purpose of the musculoskeletal system is **providing form for the body**.

**6. B**
The circulatory system is an organ system that passes nutrients (such as amino acids, electrolytes and lymph), gases, hormones, blood cells, etc. to and from cells in the body to help fight diseases and help stabilize body temperature and pH to maintain homeostasis.

**7. B**
The lungs are an important component of the respiratory system.

**8. A**
The immune system fight off disease by identifying and killing tumor cells and pathogens.

**9. D**
The primary purpose of the digestive system is to convert food into a form that can provide nourishment for the body.

**10. B**
Urine is mostly comprised of waste material after the body has taken the nutrients from food and absorbed the water it needs.

**11. A**
The gallbladder is located in the Right Upper Quadrant together with the liver, right kidney, colon, pancreas and large intestine.

**12. A**
The lymphatic system is defined as the system which carries a clear liquid lymph toward the heart.

**13. A**
The spleen is an organ found in virtually all vertebrate animals with important roles in regard to red blood cells (also called erythrocytes) and the immune system. In humans it is located in the left upper quadrant of the abdomen. It removes old red blood cells and holds a reserve of blood in case of hemorrhagic shock while also recycling iron.

**14. D**
The right upper quadrant of the abdomen, often abbreviated as RUQ, contains the liver, gall bladder, duodenum and had of the pancreas.

**15. B**
Exercise and low fat diets will increase metabolism. Choice B, **a man who is past 30 and whose body is losing muscle** is the only choice.

**16. C**
Muscle tissue can **relax and contract**, bringing out movement and the ability to work.

**17. C**
The human skin (integumentary) is composed of a minimum of 3 major layers of tissue, the Epidermis, the Dermis and Hypodermis.

**18. A**
Cartilage is a flexible connective tissue found in many areas in the bodies of humans and other animals, including the joints between bones, the rib cage, the ear, the nose, the elbow, the knee, the ankle, the bronchial tubes and the intervertebral discs. It is not as hard and rigid as bone but is stiffer and less flexible than muscle.

**19. A**
The main components of the circulatory system are the heart, veins and blood vessels.

**20. D**
The exchange of oxygen for carbon dioxide takes place in the alveolar area of the lungs.

**21. A**
Detection of pathogens can be complicated because **they evolve so quickly**.

**22. B**
Cleansing food of impurities is not an example of a function of the stomach in digestion.

**23. A**
Urea is the name of the waste removed from the body through urine.

**24. C**
An example of an organ that plays a big role in the lymphatic system is the spleen.

**25. C**
The central nervous system integrates and coordinates information from all parts of the body.

# Practice Test Questions Set 2

## Section I – Reading Comprehension

**Questions:** 35
**Time:** 60 Minutes

## Section II – Mathematics

**Questions:** 50
**Time:** 60 Minutes

## Section III English Grammar

**Questions:** 50
**Time:** 50 Minutes

## Section IV - Vocabulary

**Questions:** 50
**Time:** 50 Minutes

## Section V – Part I – Science

**Questions:** 75
**Time:** 125 minutes

## Section VI Anatomy & Physiology

**Questions:** 25
**Time:** 25 minutes

The practice test portion presents questions that are representative of the type of question you should expect to find on the HESI®. However, they are not intended to match exactly what is on the HESI®.

For the best results, take this Practice Test as if it were the real exam. Set aside time when you will not be disturbed, and a location that is quiet and free of distractions. Read the instructions carefully, read each question carefully, and answer to the best of your ability.

Use the bubble answer sheets provided. When you have completed the Practice Test, check your answer against the Answer Key and read the explanation provided.

Do not attempt more than one set of practice test questions in one day. After completing the first practice test, wait two or three days before attempting the second set of questions.

**This set of practice test questions contains all the HESI® modules. Different schools use different modules so be sure to check with your school for the modules being used.**

## Reading Comprehension

|    | A | B | C | D | E |    | A | B | C | D | E |
|----|---|---|---|---|---|----|---|---|---|---|---|
| 1  | ○ | ○ | ○ | ○ | ○ | 21 | ○ | ○ | ○ | ○ | ○ |
| 2  | ○ | ○ | ○ | ○ | ○ | 22 | ○ | ○ | ○ | ○ | ○ |
| 3  | ○ | ○ | ○ | ○ | ○ | 23 | ○ | ○ | ○ | ○ | ○ |
| 4  | ○ | ○ | ○ | ○ | ○ | 24 | ○ | ○ | ○ | ○ | ○ |
| 5  | ○ | ○ | ○ | ○ | ○ | 25 | ○ | ○ | ○ | ○ | ○ |
| 6  | ○ | ○ | ○ | ○ | ○ | 26 | ○ | ○ | ○ | ○ | ○ |
| 7  | ○ | ○ | ○ | ○ | ○ | 27 | ○ | ○ | ○ | ○ | ○ |
| 8  | ○ | ○ | ○ | ○ | ○ | 28 | ○ | ○ | ○ | ○ | ○ |
| 9  | ○ | ○ | ○ | ○ | ○ | 29 | ○ | ○ | ○ | ○ | ○ |
| 10 | ○ | ○ | ○ | ○ | ○ | 30 | ○ | ○ | ○ | ○ | ○ |
| 11 | ○ | ○ | ○ | ○ | ○ | 31 | ○ | ○ | ○ | ○ | ○ |
| 12 | ○ | ○ | ○ | ○ | ○ | 32 | ○ | ○ | ○ | ○ | ○ |
| 13 | ○ | ○ | ○ | ○ | ○ | 33 | ○ | ○ | ○ | ○ | ○ |
| 14 | ○ | ○ | ○ | ○ | ○ | 34 | ○ | ○ | ○ | ○ | ○ |
| 15 | ○ | ○ | ○ | ○ | ○ |    |   |   |   |   |   |
| 16 | ○ | ○ | ○ | ○ | ○ |    |   |   |   |   |   |
| 17 | ○ | ○ | ○ | ○ | ○ |    |   |   |   |   |   |
| 18 | ○ | ○ | ○ | ○ | ○ |    |   |   |   |   |   |
| 19 | ○ | ○ | ○ | ○ | ○ |    |   |   |   |   |   |
| 20 | ○ | ○ | ○ | ○ | ○ |    |   |   |   |   |   |

# Mathematics

|  | A B C D E |  | A B C D E |
|---|---|---|---|
| 1 | ○○○○○ | 26 | ○○○○○ |
| 2 | ○○○○○ | 27 | ○○○○○ |
| 3 | ○○○○○ | 28 | ○○○○○ |
| 4 | ○○○○○ | 29 | ○○○○○ |
| 5 | ○○○○○ | 30 | ○○○○○ |
| 6 | ○○○○○ | 31 | ○○○○○ |
| 7 | ○○○○○ | 32 | ○○○○○ |
| 8 | ○○○○○ | 33 | ○○○○○ |
| 9 | ○○○○○ | 34 | ○○○○○ |
| 10 | ○○○○○ | 35 | ○○○○○ |
| 11 | ○○○○○ | 36 | ○○○○○ |
| 12 | ○○○○○ | 37 | ○○○○○ |
| 13 | ○○○○○ | 38 | ○○○○○ |
| 14 | ○○○○○ | 39 | ○○○○○ |
| 15 | ○○○○○ | 40 | ○○○○○ |
| 16 | ○○○○○ | 41 | ○○○○○ |
| 17 | ○○○○○ | 42 | ○○○○○ |
| 18 | ○○○○○ | 43 | ○○○○○ |
| 19 | ○○○○○ | 44 | ○○○○○ |
| 20 | ○○○○○ | 45 | ○○○○○ |
| 21 | ○○○○○ | 46 | ○○○○○ |
| 22 | ○○○○○ | 47 | ○○○○○ |
| 23 | ○○○○○ | 48 | ○○○○○ |
| 24 | ○○○○○ | 49 | ○○○○○ |
| 25 | ○○○○○ | 50 | ○○○○○ |

## English Grammar

|    | A | B | C | D | E |    | A | B | C | D | E |
|----|---|---|---|---|---|----|---|---|---|---|---|
| 1  | ○ | ○ | ○ | ○ | ○ | 26 | ○ | ○ | ○ | ○ | ○ |
| 2  | ○ | ○ | ○ | ○ | ○ | 27 | ○ | ○ | ○ | ○ | ○ |
| 3  | ○ | ○ | ○ | ○ | ○ | 28 | ○ | ○ | ○ | ○ | ○ |
| 4  | ○ | ○ | ○ | ○ | ○ | 29 | ○ | ○ | ○ | ○ | ○ |
| 5  | ○ | ○ | ○ | ○ | ○ | 30 | ○ | ○ | ○ | ○ | ○ |
| 6  | ○ | ○ | ○ | ○ | ○ | 31 | ○ | ○ | ○ | ○ | ○ |
| 7  | ○ | ○ | ○ | ○ | ○ | 32 | ○ | ○ | ○ | ○ | ○ |
| 8  | ○ | ○ | ○ | ○ | ○ | 33 | ○ | ○ | ○ | ○ | ○ |
| 9  | ○ | ○ | ○ | ○ | ○ | 34 | ○ | ○ | ○ | ○ | ○ |
| 10 | ○ | ○ | ○ | ○ | ○ | 35 | ○ | ○ | ○ | ○ | ○ |
| 11 | ○ | ○ | ○ | ○ | ○ | 36 | ○ | ○ | ○ | ○ | ○ |
| 12 | ○ | ○ | ○ | ○ | ○ | 37 | ○ | ○ | ○ | ○ | ○ |
| 13 | ○ | ○ | ○ | ○ | ○ | 38 | ○ | ○ | ○ | ○ | ○ |
| 14 | ○ | ○ | ○ | ○ | ○ | 39 | ○ | ○ | ○ | ○ | ○ |
| 15 | ○ | ○ | ○ | ○ | ○ | 40 | ○ | ○ | ○ | ○ | ○ |
| 16 | ○ | ○ | ○ | ○ | ○ | 41 | ○ | ○ | ○ | ○ | ○ |
| 17 | ○ | ○ | ○ | ○ | ○ | 42 | ○ | ○ | ○ | ○ | ○ |
| 18 | ○ | ○ | ○ | ○ | ○ | 43 | ○ | ○ | ○ | ○ | ○ |
| 19 | ○ | ○ | ○ | ○ | ○ | 44 | ○ | ○ | ○ | ○ | ○ |
| 20 | ○ | ○ | ○ | ○ | ○ | 45 | ○ | ○ | ○ | ○ | ○ |
| 21 | ○ | ○ | ○ | ○ | ○ | 46 | ○ | ○ | ○ | ○ | ○ |
| 22 | ○ | ○ | ○ | ○ | ○ | 47 | ○ | ○ | ○ | ○ | ○ |
| 23 | ○ | ○ | ○ | ○ | ○ | 48 | ○ | ○ | ○ | ○ | ○ |
| 24 | ○ | ○ | ○ | ○ | ○ | 49 | ○ | ○ | ○ | ○ | ○ |
| 25 | ○ | ○ | ○ | ○ | ○ | 50 | ○ | ○ | ○ | ○ | ○ |

# Vocabulary

|     | A B C D E |     | A B C D E |
| --- | --- | --- | --- |
| 1   | ○○○○○ | 26  | ○○○○○ |
| 2   | ○○○○○ | 27  | ○○○○○ |
| 3   | ○○○○○ | 28  | ○○○○○ |
| 4   | ○○○○○ | 29  | ○○○○○ |
| 5   | ○○○○○ | 30  | ○○○○○ |
| 6   | ○○○○○ | 31  | ○○○○○ |
| 7   | ○○○○○ | 32  | ○○○○○ |
| 8   | ○○○○○ | 33  | ○○○○○ |
| 9   | ○○○○○ | 34  | ○○○○○ |
| 10  | ○○○○○ | 35  | ○○○○○ |
| 11  | ○○○○○ | 36  | ○○○○○ |
| 12  | ○○○○○ | 37  | ○○○○○ |
| 13  | ○○○○○ | 38  | ○○○○○ |
| 14  | ○○○○○ | 39  | ○○○○○ |
| 15  | ○○○○○ | 40  | ○○○○○ |
| 16  | ○○○○○ | 41  | ○○○○○ |
| 17  | ○○○○○ | 42  | ○○○○○ |
| 18  | ○○○○○ | 43  | ○○○○○ |
| 19  | ○○○○○ | 44  | ○○○○○ |
| 20  | ○○○○○ | 45  | ○○○○○ |
| 21  | ○○○○○ | 46  | ○○○○○ |
| 22  | ○○○○○ | 47  | ○○○○○ |
| 23  | ○○○○○ | 48  | ○○○○○ |
| 24  | ○○○○○ | 49  | ○○○○○ |
| 25  | ○○○○○ | 50  | ○○○○○ |

# Science

1. Ⓐ Ⓑ Ⓒ Ⓓ   21. Ⓐ Ⓑ Ⓒ Ⓓ   41. Ⓐ Ⓑ Ⓒ Ⓓ   61. Ⓐ Ⓑ Ⓒ Ⓓ
2. Ⓐ Ⓑ Ⓒ Ⓓ   22. Ⓐ Ⓑ Ⓒ Ⓓ   42. Ⓐ Ⓑ Ⓒ Ⓓ   62. Ⓐ Ⓑ Ⓒ Ⓓ
3. Ⓐ Ⓑ Ⓒ Ⓓ   23. Ⓐ Ⓑ Ⓒ Ⓓ   43. Ⓐ Ⓑ Ⓒ Ⓓ   63. Ⓐ Ⓑ Ⓒ Ⓓ
4. Ⓐ Ⓑ Ⓒ Ⓓ   24. Ⓐ Ⓑ Ⓒ Ⓓ   44. Ⓐ Ⓑ Ⓒ Ⓓ   64. Ⓐ Ⓑ Ⓒ Ⓓ
5. Ⓐ Ⓑ Ⓒ Ⓓ   25. Ⓐ Ⓑ Ⓒ Ⓓ   45. Ⓐ Ⓑ Ⓒ Ⓓ   65. Ⓐ Ⓑ Ⓒ Ⓓ
6. Ⓐ Ⓑ Ⓒ Ⓓ   26. Ⓐ Ⓑ Ⓒ Ⓓ   46. Ⓐ Ⓑ Ⓒ Ⓓ   66. Ⓐ Ⓑ Ⓒ Ⓓ
7. Ⓐ Ⓑ Ⓒ Ⓓ   27. Ⓐ Ⓑ Ⓒ Ⓓ   47. Ⓐ Ⓑ Ⓒ Ⓓ   67. Ⓐ Ⓑ Ⓒ Ⓓ
8. Ⓐ Ⓑ Ⓒ Ⓓ   28. Ⓐ Ⓑ Ⓒ Ⓓ   48. Ⓐ Ⓑ Ⓒ Ⓓ   68. Ⓐ Ⓑ Ⓒ Ⓓ
9. Ⓐ Ⓑ Ⓒ Ⓓ   29. Ⓐ Ⓑ Ⓒ Ⓓ   49. Ⓐ Ⓑ Ⓒ Ⓓ   69. Ⓐ Ⓑ Ⓒ Ⓓ
10. Ⓐ Ⓑ Ⓒ Ⓓ   30. Ⓐ Ⓑ Ⓒ Ⓓ   50. Ⓐ Ⓑ Ⓒ Ⓓ   70. Ⓐ Ⓑ Ⓒ Ⓓ
11. Ⓐ Ⓑ Ⓒ Ⓓ   31. Ⓐ Ⓑ Ⓒ Ⓓ   51. Ⓐ Ⓑ Ⓒ Ⓓ   71. Ⓐ Ⓑ Ⓒ Ⓓ
12. Ⓐ Ⓑ Ⓒ Ⓓ   32. Ⓐ Ⓑ Ⓒ Ⓓ   52. Ⓐ Ⓑ Ⓒ Ⓓ   72. Ⓐ Ⓑ Ⓒ Ⓓ
13. Ⓐ Ⓑ Ⓒ Ⓓ   33. Ⓐ Ⓑ Ⓒ Ⓓ   53. Ⓐ Ⓑ Ⓒ Ⓓ   73. Ⓐ Ⓑ Ⓒ Ⓓ
14. Ⓐ Ⓑ Ⓒ Ⓓ   34. Ⓐ Ⓑ Ⓒ Ⓓ   54. Ⓐ Ⓑ Ⓒ Ⓓ   74. Ⓐ Ⓑ Ⓒ Ⓓ
15. Ⓐ Ⓑ Ⓒ Ⓓ   35. Ⓐ Ⓑ Ⓒ Ⓓ   55. Ⓐ Ⓑ Ⓒ Ⓓ   75. Ⓐ Ⓑ Ⓒ Ⓓ
16. Ⓐ Ⓑ Ⓒ Ⓓ   36. Ⓐ Ⓑ Ⓒ Ⓓ   56. Ⓐ Ⓑ Ⓒ Ⓓ   76. Ⓐ Ⓑ Ⓒ Ⓓ
17. Ⓐ Ⓑ Ⓒ Ⓓ   37. Ⓐ Ⓑ Ⓒ Ⓓ   57. Ⓐ Ⓑ Ⓒ Ⓓ   77. Ⓐ Ⓑ Ⓒ Ⓓ
18. Ⓐ Ⓑ Ⓒ Ⓓ   38. Ⓐ Ⓑ Ⓒ Ⓓ   58. Ⓐ Ⓑ Ⓒ Ⓓ   78. Ⓐ Ⓑ Ⓒ Ⓓ
19. Ⓐ Ⓑ Ⓒ Ⓓ   39. Ⓐ Ⓑ Ⓒ Ⓓ   59. Ⓐ Ⓑ Ⓒ Ⓓ   79. Ⓐ Ⓑ Ⓒ Ⓓ
20. Ⓐ Ⓑ Ⓒ Ⓓ   40. Ⓐ Ⓑ Ⓒ Ⓓ   60. Ⓐ Ⓑ Ⓒ Ⓓ   80. Ⓐ Ⓑ Ⓒ Ⓓ

## Anatomy and Physiology

|    | A | B | C | D | E |    | A | B | C | D | E |
|----|---|---|---|---|---|----|---|---|---|---|---|
| 1  | ○ | ○ | ○ | ○ | ○ | 21 | ○ | ○ | ○ | ○ | ○ |
| 2  | ○ | ○ | ○ | ○ | ○ | 22 | ○ | ○ | ○ | ○ | ○ |
| 3  | ○ | ○ | ○ | ○ | ○ | 23 | ○ | ○ | ○ | ○ | ○ |
| 4  | ○ | ○ | ○ | ○ | ○ | 24 | ○ | ○ | ○ | ○ | ○ |
| 5  | ○ | ○ | ○ | ○ | ○ | 25 | ○ | ○ | ○ | ○ | ○ |
| 6  | ○ | ○ | ○ | ○ | ○ |
| 7  | ○ | ○ | ○ | ○ | ○ |
| 8  | ○ | ○ | ○ | ○ | ○ |
| 9  | ○ | ○ | ○ | ○ | ○ |
| 10 | ○ | ○ | ○ | ○ | ○ |
| 11 | ○ | ○ | ○ | ○ | ○ |
| 12 | ○ | ○ | ○ | ○ | ○ |
| 13 | ○ | ○ | ○ | ○ | ○ |
| 14 | ○ | ○ | ○ | ○ | ○ |
| 15 | ○ | ○ | ○ | ○ | ○ |
| 16 | ○ | ○ | ○ | ○ | ○ |
| 17 | ○ | ○ | ○ | ○ | ○ |
| 18 | ○ | ○ | ○ | ○ | ○ |
| 19 | ○ | ○ | ○ | ○ | ○ |
| 20 | ○ | ○ | ○ | ○ | ○ |

# Section I - Reading Comprehension

**Questions 1 - 4 refer to the following passage.**

**Passage 1 - The Crusades**

In 1095 Pope Urban II proclaimed the First Crusade with the intent and stated goal to restore Christian access to holy places in and around Jerusalem. Over the next 200 years there were 6 major crusades and numerous minor crusades in the fight for control of the "Holy Land." Historians are divided on the real purpose of the Crusades, some believing that it was part of a purely defensive war against Islamic conquest; some see them as part of a long-running conflict at the frontiers of Europe; and others see them as confident, aggressive, papal-led expansion attempts by Western Christendom. The impact of the crusades was profound, and judgment of the Crusaders ranges from laudatory to highly critical. However, all agree that the Crusades and wars waged during those crusades were brutal and often bloody. Several hundred thousand Roman Catholic Christians joined the Crusades, they were Christians from all over Europe.

Europe at the time was under the Feudal System, so while the Crusaders made vows to the Church, they also were beholden to their Feudal Lords. This led to the Crusaders not only fighting the Saracen, the commonly used word for Muslim at the time, but also each other for power and economic gain in the Holy Land. This infighting between the Crusaders is why many historians hold the view that the Crusades were simply a front for Europe to invade the Holy Land for economic gain in the name of the Church. Another factor contributing to this theory is that while the army of crusaders marched towards Jerusalem they pillaged the land as they went. The church and feudal Lords vowing to return the land to its original beauty, and inhabitants, this rarely happened though, as the Lords often kept the land for themselves. A full 800 years after the Crusades, Pope John Paul II expressed his sorrow for the massacre of innocent people and the lasting damage that the Medieval church caused in that area of the World.

## 1. What is the tone of this article?

a. Subjective

b. Objective

c. Persuasive

d. None of the Above

## 2. What can all historians agree on concerning the Crusades?

a. It achieved great things

b. It stabilized the Holy Land

c. It was bloody and brutal

d. It helped defend Europe from the Byzantine Empire

## 3. What impact did the feudal system have on the Crusades

a. It unified the Crusaders

b. It helped gather volunteers

c. It had no effect on the Crusades

d. It led to infighting, causing more damage than good

## 4. What does Saracen mean?

a. Muslim

b. Christian

c. Knight

d. Holy Land

**Questions 5-8 refer to the following passage.**

**ABC Electric Warranty**

ABC Electric Company warrants that its products are free from defects in material and workmanship. Subject to the conditions and limitations set forth below, ABC Electric will, at its option, either repair or replace any part of its products that prove defective due to improper workmanship or materials.

This limited warranty does not cover any damage to the product from improper installation, accident, abuse, misuse, natural disaster, insufficient or excessive electrical supply, abnormal mechanical or environmental conditions, or any unauthorized disassembly, repair, or modification.

This limited warranty also does not apply to any product on which the original identification information has been altered, or removed, has not been handled or packaged correctly, or has been sold as second-hand.

This limited warranty covers only repair, replacement, refund or credit for defective ABC Electric products, as provided above.

**5. I tried to repair my ABC Electric blender, but could not, so can I get it repaired under this warranty?**

    a.  Yes, the warranty still covers the blender

    b.  No, the warranty does not cover the blender

    c.  Uncertain. ABC Electric may or may not cover repairs under this warranty

**6. My ABC Electric fan is not working. Will ABC Electric provide a new one or repair this one?**

    a.  ABC Electric will repair my fan

    b.  ABC Electric will replace my fan

    c.  ABC Electric could either replace or repair my fan can request either a replacement or a repair.

**7. My stove was damaged in a flood. Does this warranty cover my stove?**

    a.  Yes, it is covered.

    b.  No, it is not covered.

    c.  It may or may not be covered.

    d.  ABC Electric will decide if it is covered

## 8. Which of the following is an example of improper workmanship?

a.  Missing parts

b.  Defective parts

c.  Scratches on the front

d.  None of the above

## Questions 9 – 12 refer to the following passage.

## Passage 2 - Women and Advertising

Only in the last few generations have media messages been so widespread and so readily seen, heard, and read by so many people. Advertising is an important part of both selling and buying anything from soap to cereal to jeans. For whatever reason, more consumers are women than are men. Media message are subtle but powerful, and more attention has been paid lately to how these message affect women.
Of all the products that women buy, makeup, clothes, and other stylistic or cosmetic products are among the most popular. This means that companies focus their advertising on women, promising them that their product will make her feel, look, or smell better than the next company's product will. This competition has resulted in advertising that is more and more ideal and less and less possible for everyday women. However, because women do look to these ideals and the products they represent as how they can potentially become, many women have developed unhealthy attitudes about themselves when they have failed to become those ideals.

In recent years, more companies have tried to change advertisements to be healthier for women. This includes featuring models of more sizes and addressing a huge outcry against unfair tools such as airbrushing and photo editing. There is debate about what the right balance between real and ideal is, because fashion is also considered art and some changes are made to purposefully elevate fashionable products and signify that they are creative, innovative, and the work of individual people. Artists want their freedom protected as much as women do, and advertising agencies are often caught in the middle.

Some claim that the companies who make these changes are not doing enough. Many people worry that there are still not enough models of different sizes and different ethnicities. Some people claim that companies use this healthier type of advertisement not for the good of women, but because they would like to sell products to the women who are looking for these kinds of messages. This is also a hard balance to find: companies need to make money, and women need to feel respected.

While the focus of this change has been on women, advertising can also affect men, and this change will hopefully be a lesson on media for all consumers.

**9. The second paragraph states that advertising focuses on women**

       a. to shape what the ideal should be

       b. because women buy makeup

       c. because women are easily persuaded

       d. because of the types of products that women buy

**10. According to the passage, fashion artists and female consumers are at odds because**

       a. there is a debate going on and disagreement drives people apart

       b. both of them are trying to protect their freedom to do something

       c. artists want to elevate their products above the reach of women

       d. women are creative, innovative, individual people

**11. The author uses the phrase "for whatever reason" in this passage to**

a.  keep the focus of the paragraph on media messages and not on the differences between men and women

b. show that the reason for this is unimportant

c. argue that it is stupid that more women are consumers than men

d. show that he or she is tired of talking about why media messages are important

**12. This passage suggests that**

a. advertising companies are still working on making their messages better

b. all advertising companies seek to be more approachable for women

c. women are only buying from companies that respect them

d. artists could stop producing fashionable products if they feel bullied

**Questions 13 - 16 refer to the following passage.**

**FDR, the Treaty of Versailles, and the Fourteen Points**

At the conclusion of World War I, those who had won the war and those who were forced to admit defeat welcomed the end of the war and expected that a peace treaty would be signed. The American president, Franklin D. Roosevelt, played an important part in proposing what the agreements should be and did so through his Fourteen Points. World War I had begun in 1914 when an Austrian archduke was assassinated, leading to a domino effect that pulled the world's most powerful countries into war on a large scale. The war catalysed the creation and use of deadly weapons that had not previously existed, resulting in a great loss of soldiers on both sides of the fighting. More than 9 million soldiers were killed.

The United States agreed to enter the war right before it ended, and many believed that its decision to become finally involved brought on the end of the war. FDR made it very clear that the U.S. was entering the war for moral reasons and had an agenda focused on world peace. The Fourteen Points were individual goals and ideas (focused on peace, free trade, open communication, and self-reliance) that FDR wanted the power nations to strive for now that the war had ended. He was optimistic and had many ideas about what could be accomplished through, and during the post-war peace. However, FDR's fourteen points were poorly received when he presented them to the leaders of other world powers, many of whom wanted only to help their own countries and to punish the Germans for fueling the war, and they fell by the wayside. World War II was imminent, for Germany lost everything.

Some historians believe that the other leaders who participated in the Treaty of Versailles weren't receptive to the Fourteen Points because World War I was fought almost entirely on European soil, and the United States lost much less than did the other powers. FDR was in a unique position to determine the fate of the war, but doing it on his own terms did not help accomplish his goals. This is only one historical example of how the United State has tried to use its power as an important country, but found itself limited because of geological or ideological factors.

## 13. The main idea of this passage is that

a. World War I was unfair because no fighting took place in America

b. World War II happened because of the Treaty of Versailles

c. the power the United States has to help other countries also prevents it from helping other countries

d. Franklin D. Roosevelt was one of the United States' smartest presidents

## 14. According to the second paragraph, World War I started because

a. an archduke was assassinated

b. weapons that were more deadly had been developed

c. a domino effect of allies agreeing to help each other

d. the world's most powerful countries were large

## 15. The author includes the detail that 9 million soldiers were killed

a. to demonstrate why European leaders were hesitant to accept peace

b. to show the reader the dangers of deadly weapons

c. to make the reader think about which countries lost the most soldiers

d. to demonstrate why World War II was imminent

## 16. According to this passage, catalysed means

a. analyzed

b. sped up

c. invented

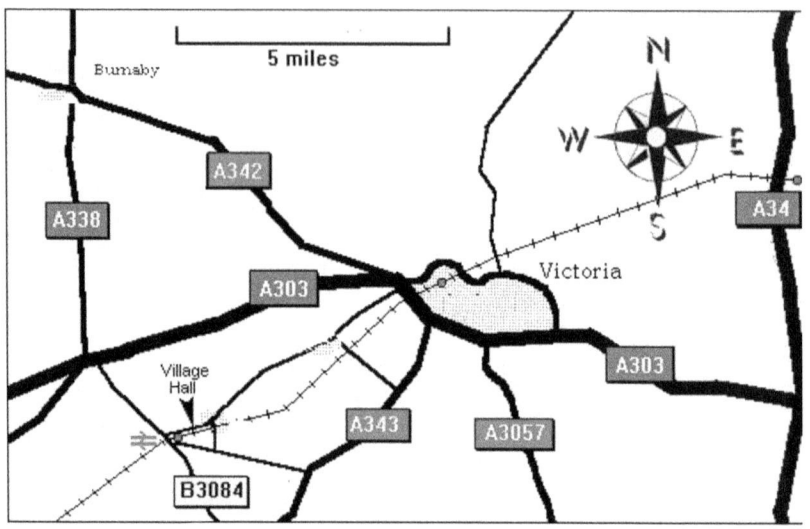

### 17. Approximately how far is Victoria to Burnaby?

    a. About 10 miles

    b. About 5 miles

    c. About 15 miles

    d. About 20 miles

### 18. How is the Village Hall from Victoria?

    a. About 10 miles

    b. About 5 miles

    c. About 15 miles

    d. About 20 miles

**Questions 19 - 23 refer to the following passage.**

**Chocolate Chip Cookies**

3/4 cup sugar
3/4 cup packed brown sugar
1 cup butter, softened
2 large eggs, beaten
1 teaspoon vanilla extract
2 1/4 cups all-purpose flour
1 teaspoon baking soda
3/4 teaspoon salt
2 cups semisweet chocolate chips
If desired, 1 cup chopped pecans, or chopped walnuts.
Preheat oven to 375 degrees.

Mix sugar, brown sugar, butter, vanilla and eggs in a large bowl. Stir in flour, baking soda, and salt. The dough will be very stiff.

Stir in chocolate chips by hand with a sturdy wooden spoon. Add the pecans, or other nuts, if desired. Stir until the chocolate chips and nuts are evenly dispersed.

Drop dough by rounded tablespoonfuls 2 inches apart onto a cookie sheet.

Bake 8 to 10 minutes, or, until light brown. Cookies may look underdone, but they will finish cooking after you take them out of the oven.

**19. What is the correct order for adding these ingredients?**

    a. Brown sugar, baking soda, chocolate chips

    b. Baking soda, brown sugar, chocolate chips

    c. Chocolate chips, baking soda, brown sugar

    d. Baking soda, chocolate chips, brown sugar

**20. What does sturdy mean?**

    a. Long

    b. Strong

    c. Short

    d. Wide

**21. What does disperse mean?**

    a. Scatter

    b. To form a ball

    c. To stir

    d. To beat

**22. When can you stop stirring the nuts?**

    a. When the cookies are cooked.

    b. When the nuts are evenly distributed.

    c. When the nuts are added.

    d. After the chocolate chips are added.

**Questions 23 - 26 refer to the following passage.**

**Passage 5 - Frankenstein**

Great God! What a scene has just taken place! I am yet dizzy with the remembrance of it. I hardly know whether I shall have the power to detail it; yet the tale which I have recorded would be incomplete without this final and wonderful catastrophe. I entered the cabin where lay the remains of my ill-fated and admirable friend. Over him hung a form which I cannot find words to describe—gigantic in stature, yet uncouth and distorted in its proportions. As he hung over the coffin, his face was concealed by long locks of ragged hair; but one vast hand was extended, in color and apparent texture like that of a mummy. When he heard the sound of my approach, he ceased to utter exclamations of grief and horror and sprung towards the window. Never did I behold a vision so horrible as his face, of such loathsome yet appalling hideousness. I shut my eyes involuntarily and endeavored to recollect what were my duties with regard to this destroyer. I called on him to stay.

He paused, looking on me with wonder, and again turning towards the lifeless form of his creator, he seemed to forget my presence, and every feature and gesture seemed instigated by the wildest rage of some uncontrollable passion.

"That is also my victim!" he exclaimed. "In his murder my crimes are consummated; the miserable series of my being is wound to its close! Oh, Frankenstein! Generous and self-devoted being! What does it avail that I now ask thee to pardon me? I, who irretrievably destroyed thee by destroying all thou lovedst. Alas! He is cold, he cannot answer me."

His voice seemed suffocated, and my first impulses, which had suggested to me the duty of obeying the dying request of my friend in destroying his enemy, were now suspended by a mixture of curiosity and compassion. I approached this tremendous being; I dared not again raise my eyes to his face, there was something so scaring and unearthly in his ugliness. I attempted to speak, but the words died away on my lips. The monster continued to utter wild and incoherent self-reproaches. At length I gathered resolution to address him in a pause of the tempest of his passion.

"Your repentance," I said, "is now superfluous. If you had listened to the voice of conscience and heeded the stings of remorse before you had urged your diabolical vengeance to this extremity, Frankenstein would yet have lived." [7]

## 23. Who is the "ill-fated and admirable friend" who is lying in the coffin?

    a. Frankenstein's monster

    b. Frankenstein

    c. Mary Shelley

    d. Unknown

**24. Why is the speaker 'suspended" from following through on his duty to destroy the monster?**

    a. The way the monster looks

    b. The monster's remorse

    c. Curiosity and compassion

    d. Fear the monster might kill him too

**25. How does Frankenstein's monster destroy Frankenstein?**

    a. By killing Frankenstein

    b. By letting himself be the monster everyone sees him as

    c. By destroying everything Frankenstein loved

    d. All of the above

**26. When the Speaker says the monster's repentance is "superfluous, what does he mean?**

    a. That it is unnecessary and unused because Frankenstein is already dead and cannot hear him

    b. That he accepts the repentance on behalf of Frankenstein

    c. That the monster does not actually feel remorseful

    d. That his repentance is unneeded because he did not do anything wrong

**Questions 27 - 30 refer to the following passage.**

**Lowest Price Guarantee**

**Get it for less. Guaranteed!**

ABC Electric will beat any advertised price by 10% of the difference.

    1) If you find a lower advertised price, we will beat it by 10% of the difference.

    2) If you find a lower advertised price within 30 days*

of your purchase we will beat it by 10% of the difference.

3) If our own price is reduced within 30 days* of your
purchase, bring in your receipt and we will refund the
difference.

*14 days for computers, monitors, printers, laptops, tab-
lets, cellular & wireless devices, home security products,
projectors, camcorders, digital cameras, radar detectors,
portable DVD players, DJ and pro-audio equipment, and
air conditioners.

**27. I bought a radar detector 15 days ago and saw an ad
for the same model only cheaper. Can I get 10% of the
difference refunded?**

    a.  Yes. Since it is less than 30 days, you can get 10%
of the difference refunded.

    b.  No. Since it is more than 14 days, you cannot get
10% of the difference re-funded.

    c.  It depends on the cashier.

    d. Yes. You can get the difference refunded.

**28. I bought a flat-screen TV for $500 10 days ago and
found an advertisement for the same TV, at another
store, on sale for $400. How much will ABC refund un-
der this guarantee?**

    a.  $100

    b.  $110

    c.  $10

    d.  $400

**29. What is the purpose of this passage?**

    a. To inform

    b. To educate

    c.  To persuade

    d. To entertain

**Questions 30 - 33 refer to the following passage.**

**Passage 6 - What Is Mardi Gras?**

Mardi Gras is fast becoming one of the South's most famous and most celebrated holidays. The word Mardi Gras comes from the French and the literal translation is "Fat Tuesday." The holiday has also been called Shrove Tuesday, due to its associations with Lent. The purpose of Mardi Gras is to celebrate and enjoy before the Lenten season of fasting and repentance begins.

What originated by the French Explorers in New Orleans, Louisiana in the 17th century is now celebrated all over the world. Panama, Italy, Belgium and Brazil all host large scale Mardi Gras celebrations, and many smaller cities and towns celebrate this fun loving Tuesday as well. Usually held in February or early March, Mardi Gras is a day of extravagance, a day for people to eat, drink and be merry, to wear costumes, masks and to dance to jazz music. The French explorers on the Mississippi River would be in shock today if they saw the opulence of the parades and floats that grace the New Orleans streets during Mardi Gras these days. Parades in New Orleans are divided by organizations. These are more commonly known as Krewes.

Being a member of a Krewe is quite a task because Krewes are responsible for overseeing the parades. Each Krewe's parade is ruled by a Mardi Gras "King and Queen." The role of the King and Queen is to "bestow" gifts on their adoring fans as the floats ride along the street. They throw doubloons, which is fake money and usually colored green, purple and gold, which are the colors of Mardi Gras. Beads in those color shades are also thrown and cups are thrown as well. Beads are by far the most popular souvenir of any Mardi Gras parade, with each spectator attempting to gather as many as possible.

## 30. The purpose of Mardi Gras is to

a. Repent for a month.

b. Celebrate in extravagant ways.

c. Be a member of a Krewe.

d. Explore the Mississippi.

## 31. From reading the passage we can infer that "Kings and Queens"

a. Have to be members of a Krewe.

b. Have to be French.

c. Have to know how to speak French.

d. Have to give away their own money.

## 32. Which group of people began to hold Mardi Gras celebrations?

a. Settlers from Italy

b. Members of Krewes

c. French explorers

d. Belgium explorers

## 33. In the context of the passage, what does the word spectator mean?

a. Someone who participates actively

b. Someone who watches the parade's action

c. Someone on the parade floats

d. Someone who does not celebrate Mardi Gras

**Questions 34 - 35 refer to the following passage.**

**Passage 7 - Peter Pan**

**Author:** James M. Barrie

All children, except one, grow up. They soon know that they will grow up, and the way Wendy knew was this. One day when she was two years old she was playing in a garden, and she plucked another flower and ran with it to her mother. I suppose she must have looked rather delightful, for Mrs. Darling put her hand to her heart and cried, "Oh, why can't you remain like this for ever!" This was all that passed between them on the subject, but henceforth Wendy knew that she must grow up. You always know after you are two. Two is the beginning of the end.

Of course they lived at 14 [their house number on their street], and until Wendy came her mother was the chief one. She was a lovely lady, with a romantic mind and such a sweet mocking mouth. Her romantic mind was like the tiny boxes, one within the other, that come from the puzzling East, however many you discover there is always one more; and her sweet mocking mouth had one kiss on it that Wendy could never get, though there it was, perfectly conspicuous in the right-hand corner.

The way Mr. Darling won her was this: the many gentlemen who had been boys when she was a girl discovered simultaneously that they loved her, and they all ran to her house to propose to her except Mr. Darling, who took a cab and nipped in first, and so he got her. He got all of her, except the innermost box and the kiss. He never knew about the box, and in time he gave up trying for the kiss. Wendy thought Napoleon could have got it, but I can picture him trying, and then going off in a passion, slamming the door.

**34. The author's description of Mrs. Darling's "sweet mocking mouth" implies:**

a. While pretty, Mrs. Darling frequently chides others.

b. Although subject to slight disfigurement, Mrs. Darling's mouth is still pleasant in appearance.

c. Mrs. Darling uses her words to get her way.

d. Mrs. Darling is a loving woman, yet she does not wholly give her love away.

**35. Overall, from this passage you can infer that Mrs. Darling:**

a. Is a dominant, complex woman.

b. Accidentally denies those around her.

c. Is artistic and absent-minded.

d. Has a troubled marriage.

# Section II – Math

**1. 8327 – 1278 =**

    a.  7149

    b.  7209

    c.  6059

    d.  7049

**2. 294 X 21 =**

    a.  6017

    b.  6174

    c.  6728

    d.  5679

**3. 1278 + 4920 =**

   a. 6298

   b. 6108

   c. 6198

   d. 6098

**4. 285 * 12 =**

   a. 3420

   b. 3402

   c. 3024

   d. 2322

**5. 4120 – 3216 =**

   a. 903

   b. 804

   c. 904

   d. 1904

**6. 2417 + 1004 =**

   a. 3401

   b. 4321

   c. 3402

   d. 3421

**7. 1440 ÷ 12 =**

   a. 122

   b. 120

   c. 110

   d. 132

**8. 2713 – 1308 =**

   a. 1450

   b. 1445

   c. 1405

   d. 1455

**9. It is known that $x^2 + 4x = 5$. Then x can be**

   a. 0

   b. -5

   c. 1

   d. Either (b) or (c)

**10. $(a + b)2 = 4ab$. What is necessarily correct?**

   a. a > b

   b. a < b

   c. a = b

   d. None of the Above

**11. The sum of the digits of a 2-digit number is 12. If we switch the digits, the number will be greater than the initial one by 36. Find the initial number.**

   a. 39

   b. 48

   c. 57

   d. 75

12. In a class of 83 students, 72 are present. What percent of student is absent?

    a.  12

    b.  13

    c.  14

    d.  15

13. Kate's father is 32 years older than Kate is. In 5 years, he will be five times older. How old is Kate?

    a.  2

    b.  3

    c.  5

    d.  6

14. If Lynn can type a page in p minutes, what portion of the page can she do in 5 minutes?

    a.  5/p

    b.  p - 5

    c.  p + 5

    d.  p/5

15. If Sally can paint a house in 4 hours, and John can paint the same house in 6 hours, how long will it take for both of them to paint the house together?

    a.  2 hours and 24 minutes

    b.  3 hours and 12 minutes

    c.  3 hours and 44 minutes

    d.  4 hours and 10 minutes

16. Employees of a discount appliance store receive an additional 20% off the lowest price on any item. If an employee purchases a dishwasher during a 15% off sale, how much will he pay if the dishwasher originally cost $450?

    a.  $280.90

    b.  $287.00

    c.  $292.50

    d.  $306.00

17. The sale price of a car is $12,590, which is 20% off the original price. What is the original price?

   a. $14,310.40

   b. $14,990.90

   c. $15,108.00

   d. $15,737.50

18. A goat eats 214 kg. of hay in 60 days, while a cow eats the same amount in 15 days. How long will it take them to eat this hay together?

   a. 37.5

   b. 75

   c. 12

   d. 15

19. Express 25% as a fraction.

   a. 1/4

   b. 7/40

   c. 6/25

   d. 8/28

20. Express 125% as a decimal.

   a. .125

   b. 12.5

   c. 1.25

   d. 125

21. Solve for x: 30 is 40% of x

   a. 60

   b. 90

   c. 85

   d. 75

22. 12 ½% of x is equal to 50. Solve for x.

   a. 300

   b. 400

   c. 450

   d. 350

23. Express 24/56 as a reduced common fraction.

   a. 4/9

   b. 4/11

   c. 3/7

   d. 3/8

24. Express 87% as a decimal.

   a. .087

   b. 8.7

   c. .87

   d. 87

25. 60 is 75% of x. Solve for x.

   a. 80

   b. 90

   c. 75

   d. 70

**26. 60% of x is 12. Solve for x.**

   a.  18

   b.  15

   c.  25

   d.  20

**27. Express 71/1000 as a decimal.**

   a.  .71

   b.  .0071

   c.  .071

   d.  7.1

**28. 4.7 + .9 + .01 =**

   a.  5.5

   b.  6.51

   c.  5.61

   d.  5.7

**29. .33 × .59 =**

   a.  .1947

   b.  1.947

   c.  .0197

   d.  .1817

**30. .84 ÷ .7 =**

   a.  .12

   b.  12

   c.  .012

   d.  1.2

**31. What number is in the ten-thousandths place in 1.7389?**

   a.  1

   b.  8

   c.  9

   d.  3

**32. .87 - .48 =**

   a.  .39

   b.  .49

   c.  .41

   d.  .37

**33. The physician ordered 100 mg Ibuprofen/kg of body weight; on hand is 230 mg/tablet. The child weighs 50 lb. How many tablets will you give?**

   a.  10 tablets

   b.  5 tablets

   c.  1 tablet

   d.  12 tablets

**34. The physician ordered 1,000 units of heparin; 5,000 U/mL is on hand. How many milliliters will you give?**

   a.  0.002 ml

   b.  0.2 ml

   c.  0.02 ml

   d.  2 ml

**35. Simplify 4³**

   a.  20

   b.  32

   c.  64

   d.  108

**36. The physician ordered 5 mL of Capacitate; 15 mL/tsp is on hand. How many teaspoons will you give?**

   a.  0.05 tsp

   b.  0.03 tsp

   c.  0.5 tsp

   d.  0.3 tsp

**37. The physician orders 70 mg morphine sulphate; 1 g/mL is on hand. How many mL will you give?**

   a. 0.05 ml

   b. 0.07 ml

   c. 0.04 ml

   d. 0.007 ml

**38. The physician ordered 200 mg amoxicillin. The pharmacy stocks amoxicillin 400 mg per tsp. How many teaspoons will you give?**

   a.  0.55 tsp

   b.  0.25 tsp

   c.  0.5 tsp

   d.  0.05 tsp

**39. The physician ordered 600 mg ibuprofen po; the office stocks 200 mg per tablet. How many tablets will you give?**

   a. 3.5 tablets

   b. 2 tablets

   c. 5 tablets

   d. 3 tablets

**40. The manager of a weaving factory estimates that if 10 machines run on 100% efficiency for 8 hours, they will produce 1450 meters of cloth. However, due to some technical problems, 4 machines run of 95% efficiency and the remaining 6 at 90% efficiency. How many meters of cloth can these machines will produce in 8 hours?**

   a.  1334 meters

   b.  1310 meters

   c.  1300 meters

   d.  1285 meters

**41. Convert 60 feet to inches.**

   a.  700 inches

   b.  600 inches

   c.  720 inches

   d.  1,800 inches

**42. Convert 25 centimeters to millimeters.**

   a.  250 millimeters

   b.  7.5 millimeters

   c.  5 millimeters

   d.  2.5 millimeters

**43. Convert 100 millimeters to centimeters.**

   a.  10 centimeters

   b.  1,000 centimeters

   c.  1100 centimeters

   d.  50 centimeters

**44. Convert 3 gallons to quarts.**

   a.  15 quarts

   b.  6 quarts

   c.  12 quarts

   d.  32 quarts

**45. 2000 mm. =**

   a.  2 m

   b.  200 m

   c.  0.002 m

   d.  0.02 m

**46. 0.05 ml. =**

   a.  50 liters

   b.  0.00005 liters

   c.  5 liters

   d.  0.0005 liters

**47. 30 mg is the same mass as:**

   a.  0.0003 kg.

   b.  0.03 grams

   c.  300 decigrams

   d.  0.3 grams

**48. 0.101 mm. =**

   a.  .0101 cm

   b.  1.01 cm

   c.  0.00101 cm

   d.  10.10 cm

**49. Smith and Simon are playing a card game. Smith will win if a card drawn from a deck of 52 is either 7 or a diamond, and Simon will win if the drawn card is an even number. Which statement is more likely to be correct?**

   a.  Smith will win more games.

   b.  Simon will win more games.

   c.  They have same winning probability.

   d.  A decision cannot be made from the provided data.

**50. How much water can be stored in a cylindrical container 5 meters in diameter and 12 meters high?**

    a.  223.65 m$^3$

    b.  235.65 m$^3$

    c.  240.65 m$^3$

    d.  252.65 m$^3$

# Section III – English Grammar

**Fill in the blank.**

**1. Elaine promised to bring the camera _____ at the mall yesterday.**

    a.  by me

    b.  with me

    c.  at me

    d.  to me

**2. Last night, he _____ the sleeping bag down beside my mattress.**

    a.  lay

    b.  laid

    c.  lain

    d.  has laid

**3. I would have bought the shirt for you if _____.**

    a.  I had known you liked it.

    b.  I have known you liked it.

    c.  I would know you liked it.

    d.  I know you liked it.

**4. Many believers still hope _____ proof of the existence of ghosts.**

    a. two find

    b. to find

    c. to found

    d. to have been found

**5. All the people at the school, including the teachers and _____ were glad when summer break came.**

    a. students:

    b. students,

    c. students;

    d. students

**6. Choose the sentence with the correct grammar.**

    a. Each player gets a locker to keep their personal things.

    b. Each player gets a locker to keep his personal things.

    c. Each player gets a locker to keep our personal things.

    d. None of the above.

**7. If he _____ the textbook like he was supposed to, he would have known what was on the test.**

    a. will have read

    b. shouldn't have read

    c. would have read

    d. had read

**8. Following the tornado, telephone poles _____ all over the street.**

    a. laid

    b. lied

    c. were lying

    d. were laying

**9. In Edgar Allen Poe's _____ Edgar Allen Poe describes a man with a guilty conscience.**

    a. short story, "The Tell-Tale Heart,"

    b. short story The Tell-Tale Heart,

    c. short story, The Tell-Tale Heart

    d. short story. "the Tell-Tale Heart,"

**10. Billboards are considered an important part of advertising for big business, _____ by their critics.**

    a. but, an eyesore;

    b. but, " an eyesore,"

    c. but an eyesore

    d. but-an eyesore-

**11. I can never remember how to use those two common words, "sell," meaning to trade a product for money, or _____ meaning an event where products are traded for less money than usual.**

    a. sale-

    b. "sale,"

    c. "sale

    d. "to sale,"

**12. The class just finished reading**
_____ **a short story by Carl Stephen-son about a plantation owner's battle with army ants.**

    a. "Leinengen versus the Ants,"

    b. Leinengen versus the Ants,

    c. "Leinengen versus the Ants,"

    d. Leinengen versus the Ants

**13. After the car was fixed, it _____ again.**

    a. ran good

    b. ran well

    c. would have run well

    d. ran more well

**14. "Where does the sun go during the _____ asked little Kathy.**

    a. night,"

    b. night"?,

    c. night,?"

    d. night?"

**15. Choose the best revision of the sentence.**

**When I was a child, my mother taught me to say thank you, holding the door open for other, and cover my mouth when yawning or coughing.**

    a. When I was a child, my mother teaching me to say thank you, to hold the door open for others, and cover my mouth when yawning or coughing.

    b. When I was a child, my mother taught me say thank you, to hold the door open for others, and to covering my mouth when yawning or coughing.

    c. When I was a child, my mother taught me saying thank you, holding the door open for others, and to cover my mouth when yawning or coughing.

d. When I was a child, my mother taught me to say thank you, hold the door open for others, and cover my mouth when yawning or coughing.

## 16. Choose the best revision of the sentence.

**Mother is talking to a man that wants to hire her to be a receptionist.**

a. Mother is talking to a man who wants to hire her to be a receptionist.

b. Mother is talked to a man who wants to hire her to be a receptionist.

c. Mother is talking to a man who wants to her. To be a receptionist.

d. Mother is talking to a man hiring her who to be a receptionist.

## 17. Choose the best revision of the sentence.

**Those comic books, which was for sale at the magazine shop, are now quite valuable.**

a. Those comics books which were for sale, at the magazine shop are now quite valuable.

b. Those comic books, which were for sale at the magazine, shop, are now quite valuable.

c. Those comic books, which were for sale at the magazine shop, are now, quite valuable

d. Those comic books, which were for sale at the magazine shop, are now quite valuable.

**18. Choose the best revision of the sentence.**

**If you want to sell your car, it's important being honest with the buyer.**

> a. If you want to sell your car, being honest with the buyer is important.
>
> b. If you want to sell your car, to be honest with the buyer is important.
>
> c. If you wanting to sell your car, being honest with the buyer are important.
>
> d. If you want to selling your car, to be honest with the buyer is important.

**19. Choose the best revision of the sentence.**

**Although today the boy was nice to my brother, they usually was quite mean to him.**

> a. Although today the boy was nice to my brother, they were usually quite mean to him.
>
> b. Although today the boy was nice to my brother, he was usually quite mean to him.
>
> c. Although today the boy were nice to my brother, he is usually quite mean to him.
>
> d. Although today the boy was nice to my brother, he were usually quite mean to him.

**20. Choose the sentence with the correct grammar.**

> a. The mother would not of punished her daughter if she could have avoided it.
>
> b. The mother would not have punished her daughter if she could of avoided it.
>
> c. The mother would not of punished her daughter if she could of avoided it.
>
> d. The mother would not have punished her daughter if she could have avoided it.

**21. Choose the sentence with the correct grammar.**

a. There was scarcely no food in the pantry, because nobody ate at home.

b. There was scarcely any food in the pantry, because nobody ate at home.

c. There was scarcely any food in the pantry, because not nobody ate at home.

d. There was scarcely no food in the pantry, because not nobody ate at home.

**22. Choose the sentence with the correct grammar.**

a. Neither of them came with their bicycle.

b. Neither of them came with his bicycle.

c. Neither of them came with our bicycle.

d. None of the above.

**23. Choose the sentence with the proper usage.**

a. Despite bad weather yesterday, he can still attend the party.

b. Despite bad weather yesterday, he could still attend the party.

c. Despite bad weather yesterday, he may still attend the party.

d. None of the above.

**24. Choose the sentence with the correct grammar.**

a. Michael has lived in that house for forty years, while I has owned this one for only six weeks.

b. Michael have lived in that house for forty years, while I have owned this one for only six weeks.

c. Michael have lived in that house for forty years, while I has owned this one for only six weeks.

d. Michael has lived in that house for forty years, while I have owned this one for only six weeks.

**25. Choose the sentence with the correct grammar.**

a. The members of the team were asked to discuss with each other.

b. The members of the team were asked to discuss with one another.

c. Both of the above.

**26. Choose the sentence with the proper usage.**

a. The man raise up quickly.

b. The man rise up quickly.

c. The man rose up quickly.

d. None of the above.

**27. Choose the sentence with the correct grammar.**

a.  He should have went to the appointment; instead, he went to the beach.

b.  He should have gone to the appointment; instead, he went to the beach.

c.  He should have went to the appointment; instead, he gone to the beach.

d.  He should have gone to the appointment; instead, he gone to the beach.

**28. Choose the sentence with the proper usage.**

a. Their wages will be rised.

b. Their wages will be rose.

c. Their salaries will be raised.

d. None of the above.

**30. Choose the sentence with the correct grammar.**

a. Every doctor must come with his stethoscope

b. Every doctor must come with their stethoscope

c. Every doctor must come with our stethoscope

d. None of the above.

## 31. Choose the sentence with the correct grammar.

a. Lee pronounced it's name incorrectly; it's an impatiens, not an impatience.

b. Lee pronounced its name incorrectly; its an impatiens, not an impatience.

c. Lee pronounced it's name incorrectly; its an impatiens, not an impatience.

d. Lee pronounced its name incorrectly; it's an impatiens, not an impatience.

## 32. Choose the sentence with the proper usage.

a. She was nodding her head, her hips are swaying.

b. She was nodding her head, her hips is swaying.

c. She was nodding her head, her hips were swaying.

d. None of the above.

## 33. Choose the sentence with the correct usage.

a. They're going to graduate in June; after that, their best option will be to go there.

b. There going to graduate in June; after that, their best option will be to go there.

c. They're going to graduate in June; after that, there best option will be to go their.

d. Their going to graduate in June; after that, their best option will be to go there

## 34. Choose the sentence with the proper usage.

a. I shall arrive early and I will have breakfast with you.

b. I shall arrive early and I would have breakfast with you.

c. I shall arrive early and have breakfast with you.

d. None of the above.

**35. Choose the sentence with the proper usage.**

    a. The tables were laid by the students.

    b. The tables were lay by the students

    c. The tables were lie by the students

**36. Choose the sentence with the correct usage.**

    a.  You're mistaken; that is not you're book.

    b.  Your mistaken; that is not your book.

    c.  You're mistaken; that is not your book.

    d.  Your mistaken; that is not you're book.

**37. Choose the sentence with the correct grammar.**

    a. The teacher asked everybody is to submit his assignment by 9 a.m.

    b. The teacher asked everybody is to submit our assignment by 9 a.m.

    c. The teacher asked everybody is to submit their assignment by 9 a.m.

    d. None of the above.

**38.  Choose the sentence with the correct usage.**

    a. He did not have to loose the race; if only his shoes weren't so lose!

    b. He did not have to lose the race; if only his shoes weren't so loose!

    c. He did not have to lose the race; if only his shoes weren't so lose!

    d. He did not have to loose the race; if only his shoes weren't so loose!

**39. Choose the sentence with the correct usage.**

a. The attorney did not want to prosecute the defendant; his goal was to prosecute the guilty party.

b. The attorney did not want to persecute the defendant; his goal was to persecute the guilty party.

c. The attorney did not want to prosecute the defendant; his goal was to persecute the guilty party.

d. The attorney did not want to persecute the defendant; his goal was to prosecute the guilty party.

**40. Choose the sentence with the correct usage.**

a. The speeches must precede the election; the election cannot proceed without hearing from the candidates.

b. The speeches must precede the election; the election cannot precede without hearing from the candidates.

c. The speeches must proceed the election; the election cannot precede without hearing from the candidates.

d. The speeches must proceed the election; the election cannot proceed without hearing from the candidates.

**41. Choose the sentence with the correct usage.**

a. Before a lawyer can rise an objection, he must first rise to his feet.

b. Before a lawyer can raise an objection, he must first raise to his feet.

c. Before a lawyer can raise an objection, he must first rise to his feet.

d. Before a lawyer can rise an objection, he must first raise to his feet.

## 42. Fill in the blank to make a correct sentence.

**Neither of the Wright Brothers _____ that they would be successful with their flying machine.**

    a.  have any doubts

    b.  has any doubts

    c.  had any doubts

    d.  will have any doubts

## 43. The weatherman on Channel 6 said that this has been the

    a.  most hottest summer on record.

    b.  most hottest summer on record.

    c.  hottest summer on record.

    d.  hotter summer on record.

## 44. Select the correct version of the sentence.

**He is a cowered person.**

    a. He is a cowardest person.

    b. He is a cowardly person.

    c. He is a coward person.

    d. The sentence is correct.

## 45. Select the correct version of the sentence.

**Why did Mr. Simpson deny to help you?**

    a. Why did Mr. Simpson refuse to help you?

    b. Why did Mr. Simpson resist to help you?

    c. Why did Mr. Simpson not accept to help you?

    d. The sentence is correct.

**46. Select the correct version of the sentence.**

**She is the most cleverest girl in the class.**

    a. She is the most clever girl in the class.

    b. She is the cleverest girl in the class.

    c. She is the most cleverer girl in the class.

    d. The sentence is correct.

**47. Select the correct version of the sentence.**

**He lived in California since 1995.**

    a. He had lived in California since 1995.

    b. He has been living in California since 1995.

    c. He has living in California since 1995.

    d. The sentence is correct.

**48. Select the correct version of the sentence.**

**Please excuse me being late.**

    a. Please excuse me for late.

    b. Please excuse my being late.

    c. Please excuse my being lateness.

    d. The sentence is correct.

**49. Choose the sentence with the correct grammar.**

    a. He doesn't have any money to buy clothes, and neither do I.

    b. He doesn't have any money to buy clothes, and neither does I.

    c. He don't have any money to buy clothes, and neither do I.

    d. He don't have any money to buy clothes, and neither does I.

**50. Choose the sentence with the correct grammar.**

a. Because it really don't matter, I don't care if I go there.

b. Because it really doesn't matter, I doesn't care if I go there.

c. Because it really doesn't matter, I don't care if I go there.

d. Because it really don't matter, I don't care if I go there.

# Section IV – Vocabulary

**1. Choose the adjective that means shocking, terrible or wicked.**

a. Pleasantries

b. Heinous

c. Shrewd

d. Provencal

**2. Choose the noun that means a person or thing that tells or announces the coming of someone or something.**

a. Harbinger

b. Evasion

c. Bleak

d. Craven

**3. Choose a word that means the same as the under-lined word.**

**He wasn't especially generous. All the servings were very judicious.**

    a. Abundant

    b. Careful

    c. Extravagant

    d. Careless

**4. Fill in the blank.**

**Because of the growing use of _____ as a fuel, corn production has greatly increased.**

    a. Alcohol

    b. Ethanol

    c. Natural gas

    d. Oil

**5. Fill in the blank.**

**In heavily industrialized areas, the pollution of the air causes many to develop _____ diseases.**

    a. Respiratory

    b. Cardiac

    c. Alimentary

    d. Circulatory

**6. Choose the best definition of inherent.**

    a. To receive money in a will

    b. An essential part of

    c. To receive money from a will

    d. None of the above

## 7. Choose the best definition of vapid.

    a. adj. tasteless or bland

    b. v. To inflict, as a revenge or punishment

    c. v. to convert into gas

    d. v. to go up in smoke

## 8. Choose the best definition of waif.

    a. n. a sick and hungry child

    b. n. an orphan staying in a foster home

    c. n. homeless child or stray

    d. n. a type of French bread eaten with cheese

## 9. Choose the adjective that means similar or identical.

    a. Soluble

    b. Assembly

    c. Conclave

    d. Homologous

## 10. Choose a word with the same meaning as the underlined word.

**We used that operating system 20 years ago, now it is obsolete.**

    a. Functional

    b. Disused

    c. Obese

    d. None of the Above

**11. Choose the word with the same meaning as the underlined word**

**His bad manners really <u>rankle</u> me.**

    a. Annoy

    b. Obsolete

    c. Enliven

    d. None of the above

**12. Fill in the blank.**

**Because hydroelectric power is a _____ source of energy, its use is excellent for the environment.**

    a. Significant

    b. Disposable

    c. Renewable

    d. Reusable

**13. Choose the best definition of torpid.**

    a. Fast

    b. Rapid

    c. Sluggish

    d. Violent

**14. Choose the best definition of gregarious.**

    a. Sociable

    b. Introverted

    c. Large

    d. Solitary

## 15. Choose the best definition of mutation.

    a. v. To utter with a loud and vehement voice

    b. n. change or alteration

    c. n. An act or exercise of will

    d. v. To cause to be one

## 16. Choose the best definition of lithe.

    a. adj. small in size

    b. adj. Artificial

    c. adj. flexible or plaint

    d. adj. fake

## 17. Choose the best definition of resent.

    a. adj. To express displeasure or indignation

    b. v. To cause to be one

    c. adj. Clumsy

    d. adj. strong feelings of love

## 18. Choose the adjective that means irrelevant not having substance or matter.

    a. Immaterial

    b. Prohibition

    c. Prediction

    d. Brokerage

## 19. Choose the adjective that means perfect, no faults or errors.

    a. Impeccable

    b. Formidable

    c. Genteel

    d. Disputation

**20. Choose the best definition of pudgy.**

    a. v. to draw general inferences

    b. Adj. fat, plump and overweight

    c. n. permanence

    d. adj. spoilt or bad condition

**21. Choose the best definition of alloy.**

    a. To mix with something superior

    b. To mix

    c. To mix with something inferior

    d. To purify

**22. Fill in the blank.**

**The process required the use of highly _____ liquids, so fire extinguishers were everywhere in the factory.**

    a. Erratic

    b. Combustible

    c. Stable

    d. Neutral

**23. Choose the best definition for the underlined word.**

**We don't want to hear the whole thing.  Just the <u>salient</u> facts please.**

    a. Irrelevant

    b. Erroneous

    c. Relevant

    d. Trivial

**24. Choose the best definition for the underlined word.**

**I don't know why he is being so nice. I am sure he has an <u>ulterior</u> motive.**

    a. Inferior

    b. Additional

    c. Simplistic

    d. Unfortunate

**25. Choose the noun that means ruling council of a military government.**

    a. Retribution

    b. Counsel

    c. Virago

    d. Junta

**26. Choose a noun that means someone who takes more time than necessary.**

    a. Manager

    b. Haggard

    c. Laggard

    d. Expound

**27. Choose an adjective that means lacking enthusiasm, strength or energy.**

    a. Hapless

    b. Languid

    c. Ubiquitous

    d. Promiscuous

**28. Choose a word that means the same as the underlined word.**

**I still don't know exactly.  That isn't <u>conclusive</u> evidence.**

a. Undeterred

b. Unrelenting

c. Unfortunate

d. Definitive

**29.  Choose the best definition of mollify.**

a. To anger

b. To modify

c. To irritate

d. To soothe

**30. Choose the best definition of redundant.**

a. Backup

b. Necessary repetition

c.  Unnecessary repetition

d. No repetition

**31. Choose the best definition of raucous.**

a. Adj. Pedantic; academic; for teaching

b. Adj. contemptuous, scornful

c. adj. Not essential under the circumstances

d. adj. harsh or rough sounding

**32. Choose the noun that means a person of influence, rank or distinction.**

 a. Consummate

 b. Sinister

 c. Accolade

 d. Magnate

**33. Choose the word that means the same as the underlined word.**

**The warehouse went bankrupt so all the furniture has to be <u>sold.</u>**

 a. Dissected

 b. Liquidated

 c. Destroyed

 d. Bought

**34. Choose the word that means the same as the underlined word.**

**He sold the property when he didn't even own it.  The whole thing was a <u>fraud</u>.**

 a. Hoax

 b. Feign

 c. Defile

 d. Default

**35. Choose the best definition of bicker.**

 a. Chat

 b. Discuss

 c. Argue

 d. Debate

**36. Choose a noun that means a lingering disease or ailment of the human body.**

    a. Treatment

    b. Frontal

    c. Malady

    d. Assiduous

**37. Choose the word that means the same as the underlined word.**

**Just because she is supervisor, doesn't mean we have to <u>cower</u> in front of her.**

    a. Foible

    b. Grovel

    c. Humiliate

    d. Indispose

**38. Choose the best definition of maverick.**

    a. Rebel

    b. Conformist

    c. Unconventional

    d. Conventional

**39. Choose the adjective that means relating to a wedding or marriage.**

    a. Nefarious

    b. Fluctuate

    c. Nuptial

    d. Flatulence

**40. Choose the adjective that means open display or apparent.**

    a. Ostensible

    b. Sign-post

    c. Revealing

    d. Harrowing

**41. Choose the word that means the same as the underlined word.**
**Her attitude was very <u>casual</u>.**

    a. Idle

    b. Nonchalant

    c. Portly

    d. Portend

**42. Choose the word that means the same as the underlined word.**
**The machine <u>powderizes</u> the rock.**

    a. Quells

    b. Pulverizes

    c. Eradicates

    d. Scgments

**43. Choose the best definition of tenuous.**

    a. Strong

    b. Tense

    c. Firm

    d. Weak

**44. Choose the noun that means a sheet of paper that can be folded into 8 leaves.**

    a. Octagon

    b. Harangue

    c. Octavo

    d. Wreckage

**45. Choose the word that means the same as the underlined word.**

**The water in the pond has been sitting for so long it is <u>dead</u>.**

    a. Stagnant

    b. Sediment

    c. Stupor

    d. Residue

**46. Choose the word with the same meaning as the underlined word.**

**She didn't listen to a thing and <u>rejected</u> all the objections.**

    a. Manipulated

    b. Mired

    c. Furtive

    d. Rebuffed

**47. Choose the best definition of pandemonium.**

    a. Chaos

    b. Orderly

    c. Quiet

    d. Noisy

**48.  Choose the best definition of perpetual.**

    a. Continuous

    b. Slowly

    c. Over a very long time

    d. Motion

**49. Choose the adjective that means appearing weak or pale.**

    a. Pallid

    b. Palliative

    c. Deviant

    d. Expatiate

**50. Choose the word that means the same as the underlined word.**
**He loaned me the money last month and is going to <u>repay</u> me tomorrow.**

    a. Reimburse

    b. Reinstate

    c. Reconcile

    d. Rebuff

# Section V – Science

**1. A soccer ball is kicked and travels at a velocity of 12 m/sec.  After 60 seconds, it comes to a stop.  What is the acceleration?**

    a.  $-0.2$ m/sec$^2$

    b.  $0.2$ m/sec$^2$

    c.  $1$ m/sec$^2$

    d.  $0.5$ m/sec$^2$

**2. A molecule of water contains hydrogen and oxygen in a 1:8 ratio by mass. This is a statement of**

    a. The law of multiple proportions

    b. The law of conservation of mass

    c. The law of conservation of energy

    d. The law of constant composition

**3. Electrons play a critical role in**

    a. Electricity

    b. Magnetism

    c. Thermal conductivity

    d. All of the above

**4.  An idea concerning a phenomena and possible explanations for that phenomena is a/an**

    a. Theory.

    b. Experiment.

    c. Inference.

    d. Hypothesis.

**5. Define chromosomes.**

 a. Structures in a cell nucleus that carry genetic material.

 b. Consist of thousands of DNA strands.

 c. Total 46 in a normal human cell.

 d. All of the above

**6. A base is**

 a. A compound that reacts with an acid to form a salt.

 b. A molecule or ion that captures hydrogen ions.

 c. A molecule or ion that donates an electron pair to form a chemical bond.

 d. All of the above are true

**7. Which disease of the circulatory system is one of the most frequent causes of death in North America?**

 a. The cold

 b. Pneumonia

 c. Arthritis

 d. Heart disease

**8. How fast is a person walking if they travel 1000 meters in 20 minutes?**

 a.  25 meters/minute

 b.  50 meters/minute

 c.  100 meters/minute

 d.  None of the above

**9. A substance containing atoms of more than one element in a definite ratio is called a(n)**

 a. Compound.

 b. Element.

 c. Mixture.

 d. Molecule.

## 10. Which of the following describes a plasma membrane?

    a. Lipids with embedded proteins

    b. An outer lipid layer and an inner lipid layer

    c. Proteins embedded in lipid bilayer

    d. Altering protein and lipid layers

## 11. Protein biosynthesis is defined as

    a. The addition of protein to foods that lack it.

    b. Ribosomes synthesizing proteins in the endoplasmic reticulum.

    c. The process of proteasomes degrading cytoplasm.

    d. Proteins "flowing" through the ER into the plasma membrane.

## 12. When we speak of separating organelles through centrifugation, we're speaking of

    a. Cell fractionation

    b. Flow cytometry

    c. Immunoprecipation

    d. Detergents

## 13. What is the difference between Strong Nuclear Force and Weak Nuclear Force?

a. The Strong Nuclear Force is an attractive force that binds protons and neutrons and maintains the structure of the nucleus, and the Weak Nuclear Force is responsible for the radioactive beta decay and other subatomic reactions.

b. The Strong Nuclear Force is responsible for the radioactive beta decay and other subatomic reactions, and the Weak Nuclear Force is an attractive force that binds protons and neutrons and maintains the structure of the nucleus.

c. The Weak Nuclear Force is feeble and the Strong Nuclear Force is robust.

d. The Strong Nuclear Force is a negative force that releases protons and neutrons and threatens the structure of the nucleus, and the Weak Nuclear Force is an attractive force that binds protons and neutrons and maintains the structure of the nucleus.

## 14. 1000 N force is applied to a concrete block that weights 500 pounds. How fast will this force accelerate the block?

a.  1 m/sec$^2$

b.  2 m/sec$^2$

c.  3 m/sec$^2$

d.  5 m/sec$^2$

## 15. What type of research deals with the quality, type or components of a group, substance, or mixture?

a. Quantitative

b. Dependent

c. Scientific

d. Qualitative

**16. When a measurement is recorded, it includes the _____ _____, which are all the digits that are certain plus one uncertain digit.**

    a. Major figures

    b. Significant figures

    c. Relative figures

    d. Relevant figures

**17. The equation $E = mc^2$ is based on the _____, and states that _____equals _____ times the _____ $^2$.**

    a. The equation $E = mc^2$ is based on the 2nd Law of Thermodynamics, and states that Mass equals Energy times (the Velocity of light)$^2$.

    b. The equation $E = mc^2$ is based on the Law of Conservation of Mass and Energy, and states that Energy equals Mass times (the Velocity of light)$^2$.

    c. The equation $E = mc^2$ is based on the 1st Law of Thermodynamics, and states that Mass equals Energy times (the Velocity of sound)$^2$.

    d. The equation $E = mc^2$ is based on the Law of Conservation of Mass and Energy, and states that the Velocity of light equals Energy times (the Mass)$^2$.

**18. Describe a pH indicator.**

    a. A pH indicator measures hydrogen ions in a solution and show pH on a color scale.

    b. A pH indicator measures oxygen ions in a solution and show pH on a color scale.

    c. A pH indicator many different types of ions in a solution and shows pH on a color scale.

    d. None of the above.

## 19. All acids turn blue litmus paper

a. Blue

b. Red

c. Green

d. White

## 20. What type of bonds involve a complete sharing of electrons and occurs most commonly between atoms that have partially filled outer shells or energy levels?

a. Covalent

b. Ionic

c. Hydrogen

d. Proportional

## 21. What can accept a hydrogen ion and can react with fats to form soap?

a. Acid

b. Salt

c. Base

d. Foundation

## 22. Which, if any, of the following statements are true?

a. Water boils at approximately 100 °C (212 °F) at standard atmospheric pressure.

b. The boiling point is the temperature at which the vapor pressure is higher than the atmospheric pressure around the water.

c. Water boils at a higher temperature in areas of lower pressure.

d. All of the above statements are true.

**23. Which gene, whose presence as a single copy, controls the expression of a trait?**

    a. Principal gene

    b. Latent gene

    c. Recessive gene

    d. Dominant gene

**24. What is the mathematical function that gives the amplitude of a wave as a function of position (and sometimes, as a function of time and/or electron spin)?**

    a. Wavelength

    b. Frequency

    c. Wavenumber

    d. Wavefunction

**25. Which of the following is not a habitat where bacteria commonly grow?**

    a. Soil

    b. The vacuum of space

    c. Radioactive waste

    d. Deep in the earth's crust

**26. Within taxonomy, plants and animals are considered two basic**

    a. Families

    b. Kingdoms

    c. Domains

    d. Genus

**27. Most of the elements on the periodic table can be classified as**

    a. Nonmetals

    b. Metals

    c. Metalloids

    d. Gas

**28. What is a chemical involved in, but not changed by, a chemical reaction by which chemical bonds are weakened and reactions accelerated.**

    a. A propellant

    b. A reagent

    c. A catalyst

    d. None of the above

**29. Organisms grouped into the _____ Kingdom include all unicellular organisms lacking a definite cellular arrangement such as _____ and _____.**

    a. Fungi, bacteria, algae

    b. Protista, bacteria, amphibian

    c. Protista, bacteria, algae

    d. Plantae, bacteria, algae

**30. Which of these statements about metals are true?**

    a. A metal is a substance that conducts heat and electricity.

    b. A metal is shiny and reflects many colors of light, and can be hammered into sheets or drawn into wire.

    c. All of the statements are true.

    d. About 80% of the known chemical elements are metals.

**31. What type of bond does a reaction of elements with low electronegativity (almost empty outer shells) with elements with high electronegativity (mostly full outer shells) create?**

    a. Hydrogen

    b. Covalent

    c. Ionic

    d. Nuclear

**32. Which of the following is not an infectious bacterial disease?**

    a. Cholera

    b. Anthrax

    c. Leprosy

    d. AIDS

**33. Define a biological class.**

    a. A collection of similar or like living entities.

    b. Two or more animals in a group, all having the same parent.

    c. All animals sharing the same living environment.

    d. All plant life that share the same physical properties.

**34. Which, if any, of the following statements about prokaryotic cells is false?**

    a. Prokaryotic cells include such organisms as E. coli and Streptococcus.

    b. Prokaryotic cells lack internal membranes and organelles.

    c. Prokaryotic cells break down food using cellular respiration and fermentation.

    d. All the statements are true.

**35. 1000 N force is applied to a concrete block that weights 500 pounds. How fast will this force accelerate the block?**

   a.  -2 m/sec²
   b.  2 m/sec²
   c.  4 m/sec²
   d.  5 m/sec²

**36. What is the process of converting observed phenomena into data called?**

   a. Calculation
   b. Measurement
   c. Valuation
   d. Estimation

**37. What law states that when two elements combine to form more than one compound, the weight of one element that combines with a fixed weight of the other are in a ratio of small whole numbers?**

   a. The Law of Multiple Proportions
   b. The Law of Definite Proportions
   c. The Law of the Conservation of Energy
   d. The Law of Averages

**38. What word describes the wide diversity of sizes and shapes found in bacteria?**

   a.  Morphologies
   b.  Cosmologies
   c.  Proteins
   d.  Spirilla

**39. The mass number of an atom is**

    a. The total number of particles that make it up.

    b. The total weight of an atom.

    c. The total mass of an atom.

    d. None of the above.

**40. Which of these statements about mechanical energy is/are true?**

    a. Mechanical energy is the energy that is possessed by an object due to its motion or due to its position.

    b. Mechanical energy can be either kinetic energy (energy of motion) or potential energy (stored energy of position).

    c. Objects have mechanical energy if they are in motion.

    d. All of the above.

**41. What three processes are involved in cell division of Eukaryotic cells?**

    a. Meiosis, mitosis, and interphase

    b. Meiosis, mitosis, and interphase

    c. Mitosis, kinematisis, and interphase

    d. Mitosis, cytokinesis, and interphase

**42. The _____ _____ of an element equals the number of protons in an atomic nucleus, and, along with the element symbol is one of two alternate ways to label an element.**

    a. Atomic unit

    b. Atomic number

    c. Atomic orbital

    d. Nuclear number

## 43. Which of the following statements, if any, are correct?

a. pH is a measure of effective concentration of hydrogen ions in a solution, and is approximately related to the molarity of H+ by pH = - log [H+]

b. pH is a measure of effective concentration of oxygen ions in a solution, and is approximately related to the molarity of O+ by pH = - log [O+]

c. pH is a measure of effective concentration of hydrogen atoms in a solution, and is approximately related to the polarity of H+ by pH = - log [H+]

d. Acidity is a measure of effective concentration of hydrogen ions in a solution, and is approximately related to the molarity of H+ by pH = - log [H+]

## 44. What chain of nucleotides plays an important role in the creation of new proteins?

a. Deoxyribonucleic acid (DNA) is a chain of nucleotides that plays an important role in the creation of new proteins.

b. Ribonucleic acid (RNA) is a chain of nucleotides that plays an important role in the creation of new proteins.

c. There are no chains of nucleotides that play a role in the creation of proteins.

d. None of the above.

## 45. How much force is needed to accelerate a car that weights 200 kg to 5 m/s²?

a.  40 N

b.  200 N

c.  1000 N

d.  1500 N

**46. What law states that every chemical compound contains fixed and constant proportions (by weight) of its constituent elements?**

    a. The Law of Multiple Proportions

    b. The Law of the Preservation of Matter

    c. The Law of the Conservation of Energy

    d. The Law of Definite Proportions

**47. Four factors that affect rates of reaction are**

    a. Barometric pressure, particle size, concentration, and the presence of a facilitator.

    b. Temperature, particle size, concentration, and the presence of a catalyst.

    c. Temperature, container material, elevation, and the presence of instability.

    d. Volatility, particle size, concentration, and the presence of a catalyst.

**48. What is the term used for bacterial species which are spherical in shape?**

    a. Bacilli

    b. Spirilla

    c. Cocci

    d. Spirochaetes

**49. A practical test designed with the intention that its results will be relevant to a particular theory or set of theories is a/an _____.**

    a. Experiment

    b. Practicum

    c. Theory

    d. Design

**50. If 3 moles of sugar is dissolved to form 2 liters of a solution, calculate the molarity of the solution.**

   a. 1 M solution

   b. 1.5 M solution

   c. 2 M solution

   d. 2.5 M solution

**51. Electricity is a general term encompassing a variety of phenomena resulting from the presence and flow of electric charge. Which of the following statements about electricity is/are true?**

   a. Electrically charged matter is influenced by, and produces, electromagnetic fields.

   b. Electric current is a movement or flow of electrically charged particles.

   c. Electric potential is a fundamental interaction between the magnetic field and the presence and motion of an electric charge.

   d. All the statements are true.

**52. Strong chemical bonds include**

   a. Dipole - dipole interactions

   b. Hydrogen bonding

   c. Covalent or ionic bonds

   d. None of the above

**53. A javelin is thrown into a field at 18 m/s. if the Javelin weighs 1.5 kg, what is the momentum?**

   a. 1.2 kg x m/s into the field

   b. 12 kg x m/s into the field

   c. 27 kg x m/s into the field

   d. 2.7 kg x m/s into the field

**54. Which of these object has greater momentum, a 2 kg truck moving east at 3.5 m/s or a 4.3 kg truck moving south at 1.5 m/s?**

    a. The first truck at 7 kg x m/s moving east

    b. The second truck at 7.45 kg x m/s due south

    c. The first truck at 6.45 kg x m/s due east

    d. The second truck at 7 kg x m/s due south

**55. What is the measure of an experiment's ability to yield the same or compatible results in different clinical experiments or statistical trials?**

    a. Variability

    b. Validity

    c. Control measure

    d. Reliability

**56. Genes control heredity in man and other organisms. This gene is**

    a. a segment of RNA or DNA.

    b. a bead like structure on the chromosomes.

    c. a protein molecule.

    d. a segment of RNA.

**57. One factor that affects rates of reaction is concentration. Which of these statements about concentration is/are correct?**

    a. A higher concentration of reactants causes more effective collisions per unit time, leading to an increased reaction rate.

    b. A lower concentration of reactants causes more effective collisions per unit time, leading to an increased reaction rate.

    c. A higher concentration of reactants causes more effective collisions per unit time, leading to a decreased reaction rate.

    d. A higher concentration of reactants causes less effective collisions per unit time, leading to an increased reaction rate.

## 58. Describe each chemical element in the periodic table.

a. Each chemical element has a unique atomic number representing the number of electrons in its nucleus.

b. Each chemical element has a varying atomic number depending on the number of protons in its nucleus.

c. Each chemical element has a unique atomic number representing the number of protons in its nucleus.

d. None of the above.

## 59. Which of the following statements about nonmetals are true?

a. A nonmetal is a substance that conducts heat and electricity poorly.

b. Most known chemical elements are nonmetals.

c. A nonmetal is brittle or waxy or gaseous.

d. All the statements are true.

## 60. The molarity of 5 liters of a salt solution is 0.5 M of salt solution. Calculate the moles of salt in the solution.

a.  2 Moles

b.  2.5 Moles

c.  2.75 Moles

d.  3 Moles

## 61. A solution with a pH value of less than 7 is

a. Acid solution

b. Base solution

c. Neutral pH solution

d. None of the above

**62. What is the distance between adjacent peaks (or adjacent troughs) on a wave?**

a. Frequency

b. Wavenumber

c. Wave oscillation

d. Wavelength

**63. An object that weighs 500 g is rolling along the road at 3.5 m/s. What is the momentum of the object?**

a. 124.9 kg x m/s along road

b. 17. 50 kg x m/s along road

c. 1750 kg x m/s along  road

d. 1.75 kg x m/s along road

**64. Is a catalyst changed by a reaction?**

a. Yes

b. No

c. It may be changed depending on the other chemicals

**65. The _____ is the prediction that an observed difference is due to chance alone  and not due to a systematic cause; this hypothesis is tested by statistical analysis, and either accepted or rejected.**

a. Null hypothesis

b. Hypothesis

c. Control

d. Variable

**66. In science, industry, and statistics, the _____ of a measurement system is the degree of closeness of measurements of a quantity to its actual (true) value.**

a. Mistake

b. Uncertainty

c. Accuracy

d. Error

**67. The horizontal rows of the periodic table are known as**

a. Groups

b. Periods

c. Series

d. Columns

**68. Which, if any, of these statements about solubility are correct?**

a. The solubility of a substance is its concentration in a saturated solution.

b. Substances with solubilities much less than 1 g/100 mL of solvent are usually considered insoluble.

c. A saturated solution is one which does not dissolve any more solute.

d. All the statements are correct.

**69. Describe a valence shell.**

a. Is the shell corresponding to the highest value of principal quantum number in the atom.

b. The valence electrons in this shell are on average closer to the nucleus than other electrons.

c. They are rarely directly involved in chemical reaction.

d. None of the above are true.

**70. To calculate the molarity of a solution when the solute is given in grams and the volume of the solution is given in milliliters, you must first**

a. Convert grams to moles, but leave the volume of solution in milliliters.

b. Convert volume of solution in milliliters to liters, but leave grams to moles.

c. Convert grams to moles, and convert volume of solution in milliliters to liters.

d. None of the above.

**71. What is the atomic number for Hydrogen?**

a. 11

b. 2

c. 1

d. 5

**72. The vertical columns of the periodic table are known as**

a. Series

b. Groups

c. Periods

d. Columns

**73. The ____ of a distribution is the difference between the maximum value and the minimum value.**

a. Distribution

b. Range

c. Mode

d. Median

**74. A cannon ball weighing 35 kg is shot from a cannon towards the east at 220m/s, calculate the momentum of the cannon ball.**

    a. 7500  kg m/s east

    b. 7700 kg m/s east

    c. 8000 kg m/s east

    d. 8500 kg m/s east

**75. Which, if any, of the following statements describing acids are correct?**

    a. An acid is a compound containing detachable hydrogen ions.

    b. An acid is a compound that can accept a pair of electrons from a base.

    c. A and B are correct

    d. None of the above

# Section VI - Anatomy and Physiology

**1. The stomach and colon are both in the**

    a. Left Upper Quadrant.

    b. Right Upper Quadrant.

    c. Right Lower Quadrant.

    d. Left Lower Quadrant.

**2. The stomach is located in**

    a. LLQ.

    b. LUQ.

    c. RUQ.

    d. RLQ.

**3. An example of something that increases a person's metabolism is**

    a. Aerobic exercise.

    b. Mental exercise.

    c. Eating a fatty diet.

    d. Reading.

**4. Nerve tissue is made up of cells known as**

    a. Neurons.

    b. Protons.

    c. Molecules.

    d. Atoms.

**5. Which sub-layer of skin gives it flexibility?**

    a. The dermis

    b. Epidermis

    c. Subdermis

    d. Dermatology

**6. What makes it sometimes difficult to diagnose an ailment within the musculoskeletal system?**

    a. Bones resist X-rays.

    b. There are no diseases associated with the musculo-skeletal system.

    c. Its close proximity to other organs within the body.

    d. Its distant proximity away from other organs within the body.

**7. One disease of the circulatory system which is often mistakenly thought to be a heart attack is**

    a. Cardiac arrest.

    b. High blood pressure.

    c. Angina.

    d. Acid reflux.

**8. An example of an important side-benefit of the respiratory system is**

    a. The air allows whistling.

    b. The oxygen expelled can be recycled for other uses.

    c. The air being expelled from the mouth allows for speaking.

    d. The air expelled from the body also expels disease and germs.

**9. The process by which the immune system adapts over time to be more efficient in recognizing pathogens is known as**

    a. Acquired immunity.

    b. AIDS.

    c. Pathogens.

    d. Acquired deficiency.

**10. A common digestive affliction that most people suffer at one time or other is**

    a. Stomach cancer.

    b. Ulceritis.

    c. Indigestion.

    d. The flu.

**11. One example of the blood stream's part in the digestive system is**

    a. Preventing infection.

    b. Carrying urea to the kidneys.

    c. Expelling the urea from the body.

    d. The blood stream has no part in the digestive system.

**12. The intestines are located in**

    a. LUQ.

    b. LLQ.

    c. RLQ.

    d. All of the above.

**13. Fluid balance is important, because the human body loses water every day through urination, perspiration, feces, and**

    a. Breathing.

    b. Resting.

    c. Meditating.

    d. Outbursts of temper.

**14. The three layers of skin are**

    a. Proton, neuron and nucleus.

    b. Epidural, Mitochondria and chromosome

    c. Inner, outer and local.

    d. Epidermis, dermis and sub dermis.

**15. An example of a minor ailment of the integumentary system is**

    a. Skin cancer.

    b. Acne.

    c. Common cold.

    d. Flu.

## 16. What is osteoporosis?

a. A brain disorder that moves to the leg bones.

b. A condition in which nerves become fragile.

c. An ailment in which muscles deteriorate.

d. An ailment in which bones become fragile because of loss of tissue.

## 17. What is a more common name for the circulatory system disease known as hypertension?

a. Anemia

b. High blood pressure

c. Angina

d. Cardiac arrest

## 18. An example of a disease of the lungs that is caused or made worse by smoking is

a. Emphysema.

b. Strep throat.

c. Muscular dystrophy.

d. Leukemia.

## 19. Which cells are an important weapon in the fight against infection?

a. Red blood cells

b. White blood cells

c. Barrier cells

d. Virus cells

## 20. Besides the kidney, the other major organ that takes part in the body's urinary system is

a. The penis

b. The Liver

c. The Stomach

d. The Bladder

**21. Which of these describes the bladder?**

a. A pea-sized, circular organ.

b. A balloon shaped, muscular organ.

c. A squarish organ about the size of the small intestine.

d. A triangular organ the same size as the heart.

**22. An example of appendages contained within the integumentary system are**

a. Lungs

b. Hair and nails

c. Nostrils

d. Ears

**23. What is an example of a serious ailment of the integumentary system?**

a. Acne

b. Skin cancer

c. Heart disease

d. High blood pressure

**24. What is a condition in which the heart beats too fast, too slow, or with an irregular beat is called?**

a. Hypertension

b. Angina

c. Cardiac arrest

d. Arrythmia

**25. What is an example of an early response by the immune system to infection?**

a. Inhalation

b. Inflammation

c. Respiration

d. Exhalation

# Answer Key

**1. A**
Choice B is incorrect; the author did not express their opinion on the subject matter. Choice C is incorrect, the author was not trying to prove a point.

**2. C**
Choice C is correct; historians believe it was brutal and bloody. Choice A is incorrect; there is no consensus that the Crusades achieved great things. Choice B is incorrect; it did not stabilize the Holy Lands. Choice D is incorrect, some historians do believe this was the purpose but not all historians.

**3. D**
The feudal system led to infighting. Choice A is incorrect, it had the opposite effect. Choice B is incorrect, though this is a good answer, it is not the best answer. The Church asked for volunteers not the Feudal Lords. Choice C is incorrect, it did have an effect on the Crusades.

**4. A**
Saracen was a generic term for Muslims widely used in Europe during the later medieval era.

**5. B**
This warranty docs not cover a product that you have tried to fix yourself. From paragraph two, "This limited warranty does not cover ... any unauthorized disassembly, repair, or modification. "

**6. C**
ABC Electric could either replace or repair the fan, provided the other conditions are met. ABC Electric has the option to repair or replace.

**7. B**
The warranty does not cover a stove damaged in a flood. From the passage, "This limited warranty does not cover any damage to the product from improper installation, accident, abuse, misuse, natural disaster, insufficient or excessive electrical supply, abnormal mechanical or environmental conditions."

A flood is an "abnormal environmental condition," and a natural disaster, so it is not covered.

## 8. A

A missing part is an example of defective workmanship. This is an error made in the manufacturing process. A defective part is not considered workmanship.

## 9. D

This question tests the reader's summarization skills. The other choices A, B, and C focus on portions of the second paragraph that are too narrow and do not relate to the specific portion of text in question. The complexity of the sentence may mislead students into selecting one of these answers, but rearranging or restating the sentence will lead the reader to the correct answer. In addition, choice A makes an assumption that may or may not be true about the intentions of the company, choice B focuses on one product rather than the idea of the products, and choice C makes an assumption about women that may or may not be true and is not supported by the text.

## 10. B

This question tests reader's attention to detail. If a reader selects A, he or she may have picked up on the use of the word "debate" and assumed, very logically, that the two are at odds because they are fighting; however, this is simply not supported in the text. Choice C also uses very specific quotes from the text, but it rearranges and gives them false meaning. The artists want to elevate their creations above the creations of other artists, thereby showing that they are "creative" and "innovative." Similarly, choice D takes phrases straight from the text and rearranges and confuses them. The artists are described as wanting to be "creative, innovative, individual people," not the women.

## 11. A

This question tests reader's vocabulary and summarization skills. This phrase, used by the author, may seem flippant and dismissive if readers focus on the word "whatever" and misinterpret it as a popular, colloquial term. In this way, choices B and C may mislead the reader to selecting one of them by including the terms "unimportant" and "stupid," respectively. Choice D is a similar misreading, but doesn't make sense when the phrase is at the beginning of the passage and the entire passage is on media messages. Choice A is literally and contextually appropriate, and the reader can understand that the author would like to keep the introduction focused on the topic the passage is going to discuss.

## 12. A
This question tests a reader's inference skills. The extreme use of the word "all" in choice B suggests that every single advertising company are working to be approachable, and while this is not only unlikely, the text specifically states that "more" companies have done this, signifying that they have not all participated, even if it's a possibility that they may some day. The use of the limiting word "only" in choice C lends that answer similar problems; women are still buying from companies who do not care about this message, or those companies would not be in business, and the passage specifies that "many" women are worried about media messages, but not all. Readers may find choice D logical, especially if they are looking to make an inference, and while this may be a possibility, the passage does not suggest or discuss this happening. Choice A is correct based on specifically because of the relation between "still working" in the answer and "will hopefully" and the extensive discussion on companies struggles, which come only with progress, in the text.

## 13. C
This question tests the reader's summarization skills. The entire passage is leading up to the idea that the president of the US may not have had grounds to assert his Fourteen Points when other countries had lost so much. Choice A is pretty directly inferred by the text, but it does not adequately summarize what the entire passage is trying to communicate. Choice B may also be inferred by the passage when it says that the war is "imminent," but it does not represent the entire message, either. The passage does seem to be in praise of FDR, or at least in respect of him, but it does not in any way claim that he is the smartest president, nor does this represent the many other points included. Choice C is then the obvious answer, and most directly relates to the closing sentences which it rewords.

**14. C**
This question tests the reader's attention to detail. The passage does state that choices A and B are true, and while those statements are in proximity to the explanation for why the war started, they are not the reason given. Choice D is a mix up of words used in the passage, which says that the largest powers were in play but not that this fact somehow started the war. The passage does make a direct statement that a domino effect started the war, supporting choice C as the correct answer.

**15. A**
This question tests the reader's understanding of functions in writing. Throughout the passage, it states that leaders of other nations were hesitant to accept generous or peaceful terms because of the grievances of the war, and the great loss of life was chief among these. While the passage does touch on the devastation of deadly weapons (B), the use of this raw, emotional fact serves a much larger purpose, and the focus of the passage is not the weapons. While readers may indeed consider who lost the most soldiers (C) when, so many countries were involved and the inequalities of loss are mentioned in the passage, there is no discussion of this in the passage. Choice D is related to A, but choice A is more direct and relates more to the passage.

**16. B**
This question tests the reader's vocabulary skills. Choice A may seem appealing to readers because it is phonetically similar to "catalysed," but the two are not related in any other way. Choice C makes sense in context, but if plugged in to the sentence creates a redundancy that doesn't make sense. Choice D does also not make sense contextually, even if the reader may consider that funds were needed to create more weaponry, especially if it was advanced.

**17. A**
Victoria is about 5 miles from Burnaby.

**18. B**
The Village Hall is about 5 miles from Victoria.

## 19. A
The correct order of ingredients is brown sugar, baking soda and chocolate chips.

## 20. B
Sturdy: strong, solid in structure or person. In context, Stir in chocolate chips by hand with a *sturdy* wooden spoon.

## 21. A
Disperse: to scatter in different directions or break up. In context, Stir until the chocolate chips and nuts are evenly *dispersed.*

## 22. B
You can stop stirring the nuts when they are evenly distributed. From the passage, "Stir until the chocolate chips and nuts are evenly dispersed."

## 23. B
Choice A is incorrect as the Monster killed Frankenstein, not the other way around. Choice B is correct, Frankenstein is dead. Choice C is incorrect - Mary Shelley is the author. Choice D is incorrect, the person is called Frankenstein.

## 24. C
The speaker 'suspended' from following through on his duty to destroy the monster due to curiosity and compassion. The other choices may seem reasonable, but are not explicitly given in the passage.

## 25. D
All the choices are correct. Frankenstein's monster destroys Frankenstein by

   a. By killing Frankenstein

   b. By letting himself be the monster everyone sees him as

   c. By destroying everything Frankenstein loved

## 26. A
Superfluous means unnecessary. Looking at the context of the word as it is used in the passage:

"Your repentance," I said, "is now superfluous. If you had listened to the voice of conscience and heeded the stings of remorse before you had urged your diabolical vengeance to this extremity, Frankenstein would yet have lived."

## 27. B
The time limit for radar detectors is 14 days. Since you made the purchase 15 days ago, you do not qualify for the guarantee.

## 28. B
Since you made the purchase 10 days ago, you are covered by the guarantee. Since it is an advertised price at a different store, ABC Electric will "beat" the price by 10% of the difference, which is,

500 – 400 = 100 – difference in price

100 X 10% = $10 – 10% of the difference

The advertised lower price is $400. ABC will beat this price by 10% so they will refund $100 + 10 = $110.

## 29. C
The purpose of this passage is to persuade.

## 30. B
The correct answer can be found in the fourth sentence of the first paragraph.

Choice A is incorrect because repenting begins the day AFTER Mardi Gras. Choice C is incorrect because you can celebrate Mardi Gras without being a member of a Krewe.

Choice D is incorrect because exploration does not play any role in a modern Mardi Gras celebration.

## 31. A
The second sentence is the last paragraph states that Krewes are led by the Kings and Queens. Therefore, you must have to be part of a Krewe to be its King or its Queen.

Choice B is incorrect because it never states in the passage that only people from France can be Kings and Queen of Mardi Gras

Choice C is incorrect because the passage says nothing about having to speak French.

Choice D is incorrect because the passage does state that the Kings and Queens throw doubloons, which is fake money.

## 32. C
The first sentences of BOTH the 2nd and 3rd paragraphs mention that French explorers started this tradition in New Orleans.
Choices A, B and D are incorrect because they are names of cities or countries listed in the 2nd paragraph.

## 33. B
In the final paragraph, the word spectator is used to describe people who are watching the parade and catching cups, beads and doubloons.
Choices A and C are incorrect because we know the people who participate are part of Krewes. People who work the floats and parades are also part of Krewes

Choice D is incorrect because the passage makes no mention of people who do not celebrate Mardi Gras.

## 34. E
There is no concrete evidence of choices A, B, or C. Choice D might be plausible, save for the fact that there are no references to birds or Mrs. Darling's trickster nature. Choice E is therefore the best answer, and the passage supports the notion that her mouth possess a special kiss that neither her daughter nor husband can attain, and in this way her mouth seems to mock them.

## 35. A
Choice A is the best-supported choice: The narrator notes, "Until Wendy came, her mother was the chief one," and further describes Mrs. Darling as a woman who will not compromise. Both Mr. Darling and Wendy are seemingly unable to access the full extent of Mrs. Darling's affection. The description of Mrs. Darling's mind as "like the tiny boxes, one within the other, that come from the puzzling East" suggests she is a woman with many layers, is impossible to understand fully, and to this end has even a foreign quality to her. B is incorrect as nothing about

her denial of her husband or daughter appears to be accidental. Choice C's "absent-minded" descriptor could be reasonable, yet "romantic" is not in this case the same as "artistic", and there is no evidence of Mrs. Darling's artistic ability. Again, in light of Mr. Darling giving up on the elusive kiss, choice D could be reasonable, however there is nothing to suggest a serious problem is present in the matrimony. Nothing suggests Mrs. Darling is indecisive, choice E is incorrect.

## Section II – Math

**1. D**
8327 – 1278 = 7049

**2. B**
294 X 21 = 6174

**3. C**
1278 + 4920 = 6198

**4. A**
285 * 12 = 3420

**5. C**
4120 – 3216 = 904

**6. D**
2417 + 1004 = 3421

**7. B**
1440 ÷ 12 = 120

**8. C**
2713 – 1308 = 1405

**9. D**
$x^2 + 4x = 5$, $x^2 + 4x - 5 = 0$, $x^2 + 5x - x - 5 = 0$, factoring $x(x + 5) - 1(x + 5) = 0$, $(x + 5)(x-1)=0$. $x + 5 = 0$ or $x - 1 = 0$, $x = 0 - 5$ or $x = 0 + 1$, $x = -5$ or $x = 1$, either b or c.

## 10. C
Open parenthesis: 2a + 2b = 4ab, divide both sides by 2 =
a + b = 2ab or a + b = ab + ab, therefore a = ab and b = ab,
therefore a = b.

## 11. B
Let the XY represent the initial number, X + Y = 12, YX =
XY+ 36, Only b = 48 satisfies both equations above from
the given choices.

## 12. B
Number of absent students = 83 – 72 = 11

Percentage of absent students is found by proportioning
the number of absent students to the total number of
students in the class = 11 * 100/83 = 13.25

Checking the answers, we round 13.25 to the nearest
whole number: 13%

## 13. B
Let the father's age=Y, and Kate's age=X, therefore Y=32+X,
in 5 years y=5x,substituting for Y will be 5x = 32+X, 5x – x
= 32, 4X=32,X= 32/8, x = 8, Kate will be 8 in 5 yrs time, so
Kate's present age = 8 - 5 = 3.

## 14. A
This is a simple direct proportion problem:
If Lynn can type 1 page in p minutes,

she can type x pages in 5 minutes

Cross multiply: x * p = 5 * 1

Then,

x = 5/p

## 15. A
This is an inverse ration problem.

1/x = 1/a + 1/b where a is the time Sally can paint a
house, b is the time John can paint a house, x is the time
Sally and John can together paint a house.

So,

$1/x = 1/4 + 1/6$ ... We use the least common multiple in the denominator that is 24:

$1/x = 6/24 + 4/24$

$1/x = 10/24$

$x = 24/10$

$x = 2.4$ hours.

In other words; 2 hours + 0.4 hours = 2 hours + 0.4 * 60 minutes

= 2 hours 24 minutes

### 16. D
The cost of the dishwasher = $450

15% discount amount = 450 * 15/100 = $67.5

The discounted price = 450 – 67.5 = $382.5

20% additional discount amount on lowest price = 382.5 * 20/100 = $76.5

So, the final discounted price = 382.5 - 76.5 = $306.00

### 17. D
Original price = x,
80/100 = 12590/X,
80X = 1259000,
X = 15737.50.

### 18. C
Total hay = 214 kg,
The goat eats at a rate of 214/60 days = 3.6 kg per day.
The Cow eats at a rate of 214/15 = 14.3 kg per day,
Together they eat 3.6 + 14.3 = 17.9 per day.
At a rate of 17.9 kg per day, they will consume 214 kg in 214/17.9 = 11.96 or 12 days approx.

### 19. A
25% = 25/100 = 1/4

**20. C**
125/100 = 1.25

**21. D**
40/100 = 30/X = 40X = 30 * 100 = 3000/40 = 75

**22. B**
12.5/100 = 50/X = 12.5X = 50 * 100 = 5000/12.5 = 400

**23. C**
24/56 = 3/7 (divide numerator and denominator by 8)

**24. C**
Converting percent to decimal – divide percent by 100 and remove the % sign. 87% = 87/100 = .87

**25. A**
60 has the same relation to X as 75 to 100 – so
60/X = 75/100
6000 = 75X
X = 80

**26. D**
60 has the same relationship to 100 as 12 does to X – so
60/100 = 12/X
1200 = 60X
X = 20

**27. C**
Converting a fraction to a decimal – divide the numerator by the denominator – so 71/1000 = .071. Dividing by 1000 moves the decimal point 3 places.

**28. C**
4.7 + .9 + .01 = 5.61

**29. A**
.33 × .59 = .1947

**30. D**
.84 ÷ .7 = 1.2

**31. C**
9 is in the ten thousandths place in 1.7389.

**32. A**
.87 - .48 = .39

**33. A**
Step 1: Set up the formula to calculate the dose to be given in mg as per weight of the child:-
Dose ordered X Weight in Kg  = Dose to be given
Step 2: 100 mg  X 23 kg = 2300 mg
(Convert 50 lb to Kg, 1 lb = 0.4536 kg, hence 50 lb = 50 X 0.4536 = 22.68 kg approx. 23 kg)
2300 mg/230 mg X 1 tablet/1 = 2300/230 = 10 tablets

**34. B**
1000 units/5000 units X 1 ml/1 = 1000/5000 = 0.2 ml

**35. C**
4 x 4 x 4 = 64

**36. D**
5 ml/15 ml kX 1 tsp/1 = 5/15 = 0.3 tsp

**37. B**
70 mg/1000 mg X 1 ml/1 = 70/1000 – 0.07 ml
(Convert 1 g = 1000 mg)

**38. C**
200 mg/400 mg X 1 tsp/1 = 200/400 = 0.5 tsp

**39. D**
600 mg/ 200 mg X 1 tablet/1 = 600/200 = 3 tablets.

**40. A**
At 100% efficiency 1 machine produces 1450/10 = 145 m of cloth.

At 95% efficiency, 4 machines produce
4 * 145 * 95/100 = 551 m of cloth.

At 90% efficiency, 6 machines produce
6 * 145 * 90/100 = 783 m of cloth.

Total cloth produced by all 10 machines = 551 + 783 =

1334 m

Since the information provided and the question are based on 8 hours, we did not need to use time to reach the answer.

**41. C**
1 foot = 12 inches, 60 feet = 60 x 12 = 720 inches.

**42. A**
1 centimeter = 10 millimeter, 25 centimeter = 25 X 10 = 250 millimeters.

**43. A**
1 millimeter = 10 centimeter, 100 millimeter = 100/10 = 10 centimeters.

**44. C**
1 gallon = 4 quarts, 3 gallons = 3 x 4 = 12 quarts.

**45. A**
There are 1000 mm in a meter, so 2000 mm = 2000/1000 = 2 meters. To divide by 1000, move the decimal 3 places to the left.

**46. B**
There are 1000 ml in a liter. 0.05/1000 = 0.00005 liters. To divide by 1000, move the decimal 3 places to the left.

**47. D**
There are 1000 mg in a gram. 30/1000 = 0.03 grams. To divide by 1000, move the decimal 3 places to the left. =

**48. A**
There are 10 mm in a cm. 0.101/10 = .0101. To divide by 10, move the decimal 1 place to the left.

**49. B**
There are 52 cards in total. Smith has 16 cards in which he can win. Therefore, his probability of winning in a single game will be 16/52. Simon has 20 winning cards so his probability of winning in single draw is 20/52.

**50. B**
The formula of the volume of cylinder is = π r²h
Where π is 3.142, r is radius of the cross sectional area, and h is the height.
So the volume will be = $3.142 \times 2.5^2 \times 12 = 235.65 \text{ m}^3$.

# Section III – English Grammar

**1. D**
The preposition "to" is correct. "To" here means give.

**2. A**
"Lie" means to recline, and does not take an object. "lay" means to place and does take an object.

**3. A**
Past unreal conditional. Takes the form,
[If ... Past Perfect ..., ... would have + past participle ... ]

**4. B**
This sentence is in the present tense, so "to find" is correct.

**5. B**
The comma separates a phrase.

**6. B**
Words such as neither, each, many, either, every, everyone, everybody and any should take a singular pronoun.

**7. D**
When talking about something that didn't happen in the past, use the past perfect (if I had done).

**8. C**
"Lie" means to recline, and does not take an object. "Lay" means to place and does take an object. Peter lay the books on the table (the books are the direct object), or the telephone poles were lying on the road (no direct object).

**9. A**
Titles of short stories are enclosed in quotation marks.

## 10. C
No additional punctuation is required here.

## 11. B
Here the word "sale" is used as a "word" and not as a word in the sentence, so quotation marks are used.

## 12. C
Titles of short stories are enclosed in quotation marks, and commas always go inside quotation marks.

## 13. B
"Ran well" is correct. "Ran good" is never correct.

## 14. D
Commas and periods always go inside quotation marks. Question marks that are part of a quote also go inside quotation marks; however, if the writer quotes a statement as part of a larger question, the question mark is placed after the quotation mark.

## 15. D
The sentence starts with a phrase, which is separated by a comma and then lists the things the speaker's mother taught, to say thank you, etc. Each item is separated by a comma.

## 16. A
When referring to a person, use "who" instead of "that."

## 17. A
The comma separates a phrase starting with 'which.'

## 18. A
"Being honest," present tense is the best choice. "The buyer" is singular so use "is."

## 19. C
The subject in the first phrase, "the boy," has to agree with the subject in the second phrase, "he is."

## 20. D
The third conditional is used for talking about an unreal

situation (a situation that did not happen) in the past. For example, "If I had studied harder, [if clause] I would have passed the exam" [main clause]. This has the same meaning as, "I failed the exam, because I didn't study hard enough."

## 21. B
In double negative sentences, one negative is replaced with "any."

## 22. B
Words such as neither, each, many, either, every, everyone, everybody and any should take a singular pronoun.   Here we are assuming that the subject is male, and so use "his." The subject could be female, in which case we would use "her," however that is not one of the choices in this case.

## 23. B
Use "could," the past tense of "can" to express ability or capacity.

## 24. D
The present perfect tense cannot be used with specific time expressions such as yesterday, one year ago, last week, when I was a child, at that moment, that day, one day, etc. The present perfect tense is used with unspecific expressions such as ever, never, once, many times, several times, before, so far, already, yet, etc.

## 25. B
When you use 'each other' it should be used for two things or people. When you use 'one another' it should be used for things and people above two.

## 26. C
The verb rise ('to go up', 'to ascend.') can appear in three forms, rise, rose, and risen. The verb should not take an object.

## 27. B
"Went" is used in the simple past tense. "Gone" is used in the past perfect tense.

**28. C**
The verb raise ('to increase', 'to lift up.') can appear in three forms, raise, raised and raised.

**29. C**
The verb raise ('to increase', 'to lift up.') can appear in three forms, raise, raised and raised.

**30. A**
Words such as neither, each, many, either, every, everyone, everybody and any should take a singular pronoun.

**31. D**
"It's" is a contraction for it is or it has. "Its" is a possessive pronoun.

**32. C**
A verb can fit any of the two subjects in a compound sentence while the verb form agrees with that subject.

**33. A**
"There" shows a state of existence. "Their" is used for third person plural possession. "They're" is the contraction of "they are."

**34. C**
The two verbs "shall" and "will" should not be used in the same sentence when referring to the same future.

**35. A**
The verb LAY should always take an object. Here the subject is the table. The three forms of the verb lay are: lay, laid and laid. The sentence above is in past tense.

**36. C**
"Your" is the possessive form of "you." "You're" is the contraction of "you are."

**37. A**
Words such as, neither, each, many, either, every, everyone, everybody and any should take a singular pronoun.

**38. B**
"Lose" is a verb meaning to misplace something or to fail at

a competition. "Loose" is an adjective meaning untied or able to move freely.

### 39. D
"Prosecute" means to begin legal proceedings against an individual or group. "Persecute" is to harass.

### 40. A
"Precede" means to go first or in front of others. "Proceed" means to go forward, or to begin something.

### 41. C
"Rise," like other intransitive verbs, is used without an object; the subject does the action on its own. For example, "The sun rises." "Raise" is a transitive verb, and is used for actions that cannot be done by a subject alone but needs an object. For example, "The student raised her hand."

### 42. C
The simple past tense, "had," is correct because it refers to completed action in the past.

### 43. C
The superlative, "hottest," is used when expressing a temperature greater than that of anything to which it is being compared.

### 44. B
"Cowardly" is an adjective used to modify a person.

### 45. A
"Deny" means to reject or disagree with the truth of something. "Refuse" means to decline to do or accept something.

### 46. B
"Cleverest" is the superlative form, and means the most clever.

### 47. B
The past perfect continuous, "has been living," is correct since the action began in the past and continues to the present.

**48. B**
"Please excuse my being late" has the same meaning as "Please excuse me for being late," and is correct.

**49. A**
Shows agreement with a negative statement by using "neither."

**50. C**
Doesn't, does not, or does is used with the third person singular--the pronouns he, she, and it. Don't, do not, or do is used with first, second, and third person plural.

# Section IV - Vocabulary

**1. B**
**Heinous:** adj. shocking, terrible or wicked.

**2. A**
**Harbinger:** n. a person of thing that tells or announces the coming of someone or something

**3. B**
**Judicious:** Having, or characterized by, good judgment or sound thinking.

**4. B**
**Ethanol:** n. a colorless volatile flammable liquid $C_2H_6O$.

**5. A**
**Respiratory:** adj. Of, relating to, or affecting respiration or the organs of respiration.

**6. B**
**Inherent:** Naturally a part or consequence of something.

**7. A**
**Vapid:** adj. tasteless or bland.

**8. C**
**Waif:** n. homeless child or stray.

**9. D**
**Homologous:** adj. similar or identical.

**10. B**
**Obsolete:** adj. no longer in use; gone into disuse; disused or neglected.

**11. A**
**Rankle:** v. To cause irritation or deep bitterness.

**12. D**
**Reusable**

**13. C**
**Torpid:** adj. Lazy, lethargic or apathetic.

**14. A**
**Gregarious:** adj. Describing one who enjoys being in crowds and socializing.

**15. B**
**Mutation:** n. a change or alteration.

**16. C**
**Lithe:** adj. flexible or pliant.

**17. A**
**Resent:** v. to express displeasure or indignation.

**18. A**
**Immaterial:** adj. irrelevant not having substance or matter.

**19. A**
**Impeccable:** adj. perfect, no faults or errors.

**20. B**
**Pudgy:** adj. fat, plump or overweight.

**21. C**
**Alloy:** v. Mix or combine; often used of metals.

**22. B**
**Combustible:** adj. Able to catch fire and burn easily.

**23. C**
**Salient:** adj. Worthy of note; pertinent or relevant.

**24. B**
**Ulterior:** adj. beyond what is obvious or evident.

**25. D**
**Junta:** n. ruling council of a military government.

**26. C**
**Laggard:** n. someone who takes more time than necessary.

**27. B**
**Languid:** adj. lacking enthusiasm, strength or energy.

**28. D**
**Conclusive:** adj. Providing an end to something; decisive.

**29. D**
**Mollify:** v. To ease a burden; make less painful; to comfort.

**30. C**
**Redundant:** adj.  Unnecessary repetition.

**31. D**
**Raucous:** adj. harsh or rough sounding.

**32. D**
**Magnate:** n. a person of influence, rank or distinction.

**33. B**
**Liquidate:** v. to convert assets into cash.

**34. A**
**Hoax:** n. To deceive (someone) by making them believe something which has been maliciously or mischievously fabricated.

**35. C**
**Bicker:** n. To quarrel in a tiresome, insulting manner.

**36. C**
**Malady:** n. A disease or ailment.

**37. B**
**Grovel:** To abase oneself before another person.

**38. A**
**Maverick:** n. Showing independence in thoughts or actions.

**39. C**
**Nuptial:** adj. Of or pertaining to wedding and marriage.

**40. A**
**Ostensible:** adj. meant for open display; apparent.

**41. B**
**Nonchalant:** adj. Casually calm and relaxed.

**42. B**
**Pulverize:** v. to completely destroy, especially by crushing to fragments or a powder.

**43. D**
**Tenuous:** adj. Thin in substance or consistency.

**44. C**
**Octavo:** n. A sheet of paper 7 to 10 inches high and 4.5 to 6 inches wide, the size varying with the large original sheet used to create it. Made by folding the original sheet three times to produce eight leaves.

**45. A**
**Stagnant:** adj. lacking freshness, motion, flow, progress, or change; stale; motionless; still.

**46. D**
**Rebuff:** n. a sudden resistance or refusal.

**47. A**
**Pandemonium:** n. Chaos; tumultuous or lawless violence.

**48. A**
**Perpetual:** adj. Continuing uninterrupted.

**49. A**
**Pallid:** adj. Appearing weak, pale, or wan.

**50. A**
**Reimburse:** v. To compensate with pay or money; especially, to repay money spent on one's behalf.

# Section V – Science

**1. A**
The formula for acceleration = $A = (V_f - V_0)/t$
so $A = (0 - 12)/60$ sec $= -0.2$ m/sec$^2$

**2. A**
The Law of Multiple Proportions states that when two elements combine to form more than one compound, the weights of one element that combine with a fixed weight of the other are in a ratio of small whole numbers.

**3. D**
All of the above are true. Electrons play an essential role in electricity, magnetism, and thermal conductivity.

**4. D**
An idea concerning a phenomena and possible explanations for that phenomena is an hypothesis.

## 5. D
All of the above. Chromosomes are

    a. Structures in a cell nucleus that carry genetic material.
    b. Consist of thousands of DNA strands.
    c. Total 46 in a normal human cell.

## 6. D
All the statements about bases are true.

    a. A compound that reacts with an acid to form a salt.

    b. A molecule or ion that captures hydrogen ions.

    c. A molecule or ion that donates an electron pair to form a chemical bond.

## 7. D
The circulatory system disease that is one of the most frequent causes of death in North America is heart disease.

## 8. B
Speed = (total distance traveled)/(total time taken)
X = 1000m/20 minutes
X = 50 meters

## 9. A
A chemical compound is a chemical substance comprising atoms from two or more elements in a specific ration as expressed in the chemical formula i.e., H2O

## 10. C
The plasma membrane or cell membrane protects the cell from outside forces. It consists of the lipid bilayer with embedded proteins

## 11. C
Protein biosynthesis is defines as, ribosomes synthesizing proteins in the endoplasmic reticulum. This process, also known as protein biosynthesis, is a process within the cell by which the substrates convert to products of higher complexity.

## 12. A
Cell fractionation. Fractionation is important because it purifies the cell and its parts.

**13. A**

The Strong Nuclear Force is an attractive force that binds protons and neutrons and maintains the structure of the nucleus, and the Weak Nuclear Force is responsible for the radioactive beta decay and other subatomic reactions.

**14. B**

Force = Mass times Acceleration Measured in Newtons.
1000 = 500 x A
A = 1000/500 = 2 m/s$^2$

**15. D**

Qualitative research deals with the quality, type or components of a group, substance, or mixture.

**16. B**

When a measurement is recorded, it includes the significant figures, which are all the digits that are certain plus one uncertain digit.

**17. B**

The equation E = mc$^2$ is based on the Law of Conservation of Mass and Energy, and     states that Energy equals Mass times the Velocity of light.

**18. A**

A pH indicator measures hydrogen ions in a solution and show pH on a color scale.

**19. B**

Acids turns blue litmus paper red, base turns red litmus paper blue.

**20. A**

Covalent bonds involve a complete sharing of electrons and occurs most commonly between atoms that have partially filled outer shells or energy levels.

**21. C**

A base is any substance that can accept a hydrogen ion and can react with fats to form soap.

**22. A**

Water boils at approximately 100 °C (212 °F) at standard atmospheric pressure.

**23. D**
The dominant gene controls the expression of a trait.

**24. D**
Wavefunction is a mathematical function that gives the amplitude  of a wave as a function of position (and sometimes, as a function of time and/or electron spin).

**Note:** Wavefunctions are used in chemistry to represent the behavior of electrons bound in atoms or molecules.

**25. B**
The vacuum of space is an environment where bacteria do not commonly exit. The nature of outer space, including intense cold and lack of oxygen, makes it difficult for even most bacteria to grow.

**26. B**
Plants and animals are kingdoms.  There are six recognized kingdoms:  Animalia, Plantae, Protista, Fungi, Bacteria, and Archaea.

**27. B**
The elements on the periodic table can be classified as metals, metalloids and non-metals. Most of the elements on the table can be classified as metals.

**28. C**
A catalyst is a chemical involved in, but not changed by, a chemical reaction by which chemical bonds are weakened and reactions accelerated.

**29. C**
Organisms grouped into the **Protista** Kingdom include all unicellular organisms lacking a definite cellular arrangement such as **bacteria** and **algae.**

**30. C**
All the statements are true.

> A metal is a substance that conducts heat and electricity.
>
> A metal is shiny and reflects many colors of light, and can be hammered into sheets or drawn into wire.
>
> About 80% of the known chemical elements are metals.

**31. C**
The reaction of elements with low electronegativity(almost empty outer shells) with elements with high electronegativity (mostly full outer shells) gives rise to Ionic bonds.

**32. D**
AIDS (or Acquired Immune Deficiency Syndrome) is carried by a virus, not bacteria.

**33. A**
A collection of similar or like living entities. Class has the same meaning in biology as rank. Common classes or ranks include species, order, and phylum.

**34. D**
All the statements are true.

> a. Prokaryotic cells include such organisms as E. coli and Streptococcus.
>
> b. Prokaryotic cells lack internal membranes and organelles.
>
> c. Prokaryotic cells break down food using cellular respiration and fermentation.

**35. B**
Force = Mass times Acceleration Measured in Newtons.
1000 = 500 x A
A = 1000/500 = 2 m/s$^2$

**36. B**
The process of converting observed phenomena into data is called measurement.

**37. A**
The Law of Multiple Proportions states that when two elements combine to form more than one compound, the weights of one element that combine with a fixed weight of the other are in a ratio of small whole numbers.

**38. A**
Morphology is the field that studies the relationship between structures in living organisms.

**39. A**
The mass number of an atom is the total number of particles (protons and neutrons) that make it up.

## 40. A
All the statements are true.

a. Mechanical energy is the energy that is possessed by an object due to its motion or due to its position.

b. Mechanical energy can be either kinetic energy (energy of motion) or potential energy (stored energy of position).

c. Objects have mechanical energy if they are in motion

## 41. D
In Eukaryotic cells, the cell cycle is the cycle of events involving cell division, including mitosis, cytokinesis, and interphase.

## 42. B
The atomic number of an element equals the number of protons in an atomic nucleus, and, along with the element symbol is one of two alternate ways to label an element.

## 43. A
pH is a measure of effective concentration of hydrogen ions in a solution, and is approximately related to the molarity of H+ by pH = - log [H+]

## 44. B
Ribonucleic acid (RNA) is a chain of nucleotides that plays an important role in the creation of new proteins.

## 45. C
Force = Mass times Acceleration Measured in Newtons.
F = 200 X 5 = 1000 N

## 46. D
The Law of Definite Proportions states that every chemical compound contains fixed and constant proportions (by weight) of its constituent elements.

## 47. B
Four factors that affect rates of reaction are: Temperature, particle size, concentration, and the presence of a catalyst.

## 48. C
Spherical bacteria are Cocci. Along with bacilli, this is one of the two major structures for bacteria.

**49. A**
A practical test designed with the intention that its results will be relevant to a particular theory or set of theories is an experiment.

**50. B**
The formula for calculating molarity when the moles of the solute and liters of the solution are given is = moles of solute/ liters of solution.
Moles of Solute = 3 moles of sugar
Solution liters = 3 liters
Molarity of solution = ?

Therefore: molarity of the solution = 3 moles of solvent/ 2 liters of solution = 1.5 M solution.

**51. D**
All the statements are true.

a. Electrically charged matter is influenced by, and produces, electromagnetic fields.

b. Electric current is a movement or flow of electrically charged particles.

c. Electric potential is a fundamental interaction between the magnetic field and the presence and motion of an electric charge.

**52. C**
Covalent or ionic bonds are considered "strong bonds."

**53. C**
P = 1.5 x 18 = 27 kg x m/s into the field.

**54. A**
Momentum of first object = 2 x 3.5 = 7; momentum of second truck = 4.3 x 1.5 = 6.45. First truck has more momentum at 7 kg x m/s moving east.

**55. D**
Reliability refers to the measure of an experiment's ability to yield the same or compatible results in different clinical experiments or statistical trials.

**56. A**
Genes are made from a long molecule called DNA, which is copied and inherited across generations. DNA is made of

simple units that line up in a particular order within this large molecule. The order of these units carries genetic information, similar to how the order of letters on a page carries information. The language used by DNA is called the genetic code, which lets organisms read the information in the genes. This information is the instructions for constructing and operating a living organism.

### 57. A
A higher concentration of reactants causes more effective collisions per unit time, leading to an increased reaction rate.

### 58. C
Each chemical element has a unique atomic number representing the number of protons in its nucleus.

### 59. D
All the statements are about non-metals are true.

a. A nonmetal is a substance that conducts heat and electricity poorly.

b. Most known chemical elements are nonmetals.

c. A nonmetal is brittle or waxy or gaseous.

### 60. B
Moles of solute = ? or X
Solutions liters = 5 liters
Molarity of solution = 0.5 M

Therefore:   X moles/5 liters of solution = 0.5 or X/5 = 0.5
So X = 5/0.5
X = 2.5
Mole of salt in the solution is 2.5 moles

### 61. A
A solution with a pH value of less than 7 is acid.  A pH value of 7 is neutral.

### 62. D
Wavelength is defined as the distance between adjacent peaks (or adjacent troughs) on a wave.

**Note:**  Varying the wavelength of light changes its color; varying the wavelength of sound changes its pitch.

## 63. D
First convert 500 g to kg = 500/1000 = 0.5 kg, momentum = 0.5 x 3.5 = 1.75 kg x m/s along the road.

## 64. B
A catalyst is never changed in a chemical reaction.

## 65. A
The prediction that an observed difference is due to chance alone and not due to a systematic cause; this hypothesis is tested by statistical analysis, and accepted or rejected is the **null hypothesis**.

## 66. C
In science and engineering, the **accuracy** of a measurement system is the degree of  closeness of measurements of a quantity to its actual (true) value.

## 67. B
The horizontal rows from right to left of the periodic table are known as periods and elements on a row share the same number of electron shells.

## 68. D
All the statements about solubility are correct.

a. The solubility of a substance is its concentration in a saturated solution.

b. Substances with solubilities much less than 1 g/100 mL of solvent are usually considered insoluble.

c. A saturated solution is one which does not dissolve any more solute.

## 69. A
A valence shell is the shell corresponding to the highest value of principal quantum number in the atom.

## 70. C
To calculate the Molarity of a solution when the solute is given in grams and the volume of the solution is given in milliliters, you must first **convert grams to moles, and convert volume of solution in milliliters to liters.**

**71. C**
Hydrogen is the first element listed on the periodic table. The atomic number for hydrogen is 1.

**72. B**
Vertical columns on the periodic table are called groups. There are 18 groups on the table. Elements in the same group have the same number of electrons on their outermost shell.

**73. B**
The **range** of a distribution is the difference between the maximum value and the minimum value.

**74. B**
Formula - P = kg x m/s
= 35kg x 220 m/s
= 7700 kg x m/s east

**75. C**
A and B are correct.
An acid is a compound containing detachable hydrogen ions.
An acid is a compound that can accept a pair of electrons from a base.

# Section VI – Anatomy and Physiology

**1. A**
The stomach and colon are both in the Left Upper Quadrant, together with, liver, spleen, left kidney, pancreas and large intestine.

**2. B**
The stomach and colon are both in the Left Upper Quadrant, together with, liver, spleen, left kidney, pancreas and large intestine.

**3. A**
Exercise will increase metabolism.

**4. A**
Nerve tissue is made up of cells known as neurons.

**5. D**
The dermis, which contains Collagen and Elastin, gives skin its flexibility.

**6. C**
It is difficult to diagnose an ailment within the musculoskeletal system because of its close proximity to other organs within the body.

**7. C**
Angina is a severe pain in the chest that results from a lack of blood, therefore oxygen supply to the heart muscle.

**8. C**
An important side-benefit of the respiratory system is the air being expelled from the mouth allows for speaking.

**9. A**
The process by which the immune system adapts over time to be more efficient in recognizing pathogens is known as acquired immunity.

**10. C**
Indigestion is a common digestive affliction that most people suffer at one time or other.

**11. B**
Carrying urea to the kidneys is one example of the blood stream's part in the digestive system.

**12. D**
All of the above. The Large Intestine passes through all the quadrants.

**13. A**
Fluid balance is important, because the human body loses water every day through urination, perspiration, feces, and breathing.

**14. D**
The human skin (integumentary) is composed of a minimum of 3 major layers of tissue, the Epidermis, the Dermis and Hypodermis.

**15. B**
Acne is an example of a minor ailment of the integumentary system.

**16. D**
Osteoporosis is a disease of the bones that which increases the risk of fracture and breaks.

**17. B**
High blood pressure is a more common name for the circulatory system disease known as hypertension. Hypertension (HTN) or high blood pressure is a cardiac chronic medical condition in which the systemic arterial blood pressure is elevated.

**18. A**
Emphysema is a disease of the lungs that cause shortness of breath.

**19. B**
White blood cells are an important weapon in the fight against infection.

**20. D**
Besides the kidney, the other major organ that takes part in the body's urinary system is the bladder.

**21. B**
The bladder is a balloon shaped, muscular organ.

**22. B**
The appendages of the integumentary system are hair, scales, feathers, and nails.

**23. B**
Skin cancer is an example of a serious ailment of the integumentary system.

**24. D**
Cardiac dysrhythmia (also called irregular heartbeat or arrhythmia) describes a group of conditions where there is abnormal electrical activity in the heart.

**25. B**
Inflammation is an example of an early response by the immune system to infection.

# Conclusion

CONGRATULATIONS! You have made it this far because you have applied yourself diligently to practicing for the exam and no doubt improved your potential score considerably! Getting into a good school is a huge step in a journey that might be challenging at times but will be many times more rewarding and fulfilling. That is why being prepared is so important.

Study then Practice and then Succeed!

**Good Luck!**

## Register for Free Updates and More Practice Test Questions

Register your purchase at https://www.test-preparation.ca/register/ for fast and convenient access to updates, errata, free test tips and more practice test questions.

# HESI Test Strategy

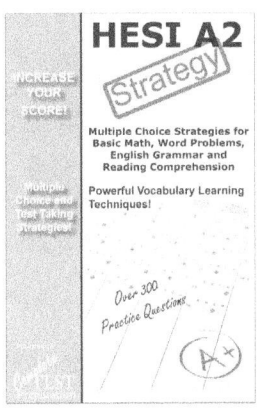

Learn and Practice Proven multiple choice strategies for Reading Comprehension, Word Problems, English Grammar and Basic Math!

If you are preparing for the Health Education Systems Exam, you probably want all the help you can get! HESI Test Strategy is your complete guide to answering multiple choice questions!

You will learn:

- Powerful multiple choice strategies with practice questions - Learn 15 powerful multiple choice strategies and then practice.

- How to prepare for a multiple choice exam

- Who does well on multiple choice exams and who does not - and how to make sure you do!

- How to handle trick questions

- Step-by-step strategy for answering multiple choice - on any subject!

- Common Mistakes on a Test - and how to avoid them

- How to avoid test anxiety

- How to prepare for a test - proper preparation for your exam will definitely boost your score!

**https://www.test-preparation.ca/hesi-strategy/**

www.ingramcontent.com/pod-product-compliance
Lightning Source LLC
Chambersburg PA
CBHW051448170526
45166CB00001B/166